WHAT NOURISHES US

How mindful eating can help us get healthy, feel well and connect with ourselves and others.

The latest insights into the holistic medicine of nutrition

DR GREGOR HASLER

Translation from the German
by
Ayça Türkoğlu

MERCIER PRESS

MERCIER PRESS
Cork
www.mercierpress.ie

Original title: *Was uns wirklich nährt*, by Gregor Hasler
© 2024 by Arkana, a division of Penguin Random House Verlagsgruppe GmbH, München, Germany.

First published in English by Mercier Press, 2026

© Translation from the German, Ayça Türkoğlu
Edited by Dr Janette Walton

ISBN: 9781806900022

eBook:9781806900039

Large Print Edition: 9781806900497

Cover design: Nord Compo

Printed and bound in the EU.

Contents

Note

This book should not be used as a medical guide in the purest sense, although its contents are reliable and could be useful. If serious illness is suspected, medical help should be sought immediately. The publisher can accept no responsibility for any consequences of the advice given here, for any illness caused by the practice of the techniques described, or for any prosecution relating to the treatment of people that may arise directly or indirectly from the information described in this book. The reader should assume full responsibility for any practical use of the information provided. If in doubt, consult a medical practitioner.

Introduction

Food is far more than the sum of its nutrients. While nutritional science has, quite rightly, devoted decades to understanding the roles of protein, fats, carbohydrates, vitamins and minerals in human health, eating itself is not a purely biochemical act. Food carries meaning. It conveys comfort, celebration, identity and a sense of belonging. It is shaped by memory and emotion, by social expectation and habit and by the physical and cultural environments in which we live. As a nutritional scientist who has spent over thirty years teaching and researching the role of diet across the life course, I have come to appreciate that any meaningful discussion of eating must move beyond nutrients on a page and engage with the lived experience of food.

In Ireland, this lived experience is deeply embedded in culture and history. Food has long been central to Irish social life – from the shared family meal to the ritual of tea and conversation, from festive occasions to moments of comfort in times of hardship. Traditional food practices evolved in response to geography, climate and agricultural systems, shaping diets that were once largely seasonal and locally sourced. Although the Irish food system has transformed dramatically in recent decades, food remains a powerful social currency. Eating is rarely a solitary act; it is woven into our relationships, our routines and our sense of place. Any attempt to understand food choice, therefore, must take account of these cultural dimensions alongside biological need.

Yet contemporary eating in Ireland takes place in a vastly different context from that of previous generations. Globalised food supply chains, modern retail environments and increasingly busy lifestyles have reshaped how food is accessed, prepared and consumed. National dietary surveys in Ireland (of which I am a lead investigator), including the National Adult Nutrition Survey (NANS) and successive child and adolescent surveys, provide a detailed picture of these changes over time (www.iuna.net). They show a pattern of diets characterised by high availability of energy-dense, nutrient-poor foods alongside persistently low intakes of dietary fibre, whole grains, fruits and vegetables in many population groups. These patterns are not simply the result of individual choice or lack of nutritional knowledge; they reflect an environment that powerfully influences what and how we eat.

At the heart of eating behaviour lie two closely related but distinct drivers: hunger and appetite. Hunger and appetite are often used interchangeably, but they describe different processes. Hunger is a physiological signal. It reflects the body's need for energy and nutrients and is regulated by complex interactions between hormones, the nervous system and metabolic demands. Hunger builds gradually and, if ignored, becomes harder to dismiss. Appetite, by contrast, is mainly psychological and sensory. It is shaped by sight, smell, memory, emotion and context. One can have a strong appetite without being physically hungry, and genuine hunger with little appetite at all. In today's Irish food environment, where palatable foods are abundant, affordable and heavily marketed, appetite is frequently stimulated in the absence of true physiological hunger.

This distinction becomes clear in everyday life. We may feel full (and without hunger) after a substantial dinner, yet still desire and have room for a dessert or something sweet. The desire is driven by pleasure, familiarity and social cues rather than bodily need. Equally, an older person living alone may experience hunger but little appetite, especially if eating has become a solitary or joyless task. The body asks for nourishment, but the motivation to eat is weak.

Appetite is often closely tied to social ritual. Many people will report not being hungry until dinner is on the table, at which point appetite suddenly appears. The smell of rashers in the morning, the sight of a roast on a Sunday, or the offer of tea and biscuits during a visit can all stimulate appetite, regardless of hunger. Neither hunger nor appetite is inherently good or bad. Understanding what drives our desire to eat helps us respond more wisely and with greater self-trust. Analyses from our dietary surveys in Ireland indicate that while health is recognised as an important determinant of food choice, taste, convenience and habit frequently exert a more substantial influence on what people actually eat. These findings reinforce the idea that eating is rarely a purely rational or nutritionally driven act.

In this context, mindful eating becomes particularly relevant. Mindful eating is not a diet, nor is it a rejection of cultural food practices. Instead, it is an approach that encourages deliberate, non-judgemental awareness of the eating experience. It involves paying attention to internal cues of hunger and fullness, to the sensory qualities of food, and to the emotional and environmental factors that shape eating behaviour. Importantly, mindful eating invites reflection rather than restriction. It asks not 'Should I eat this?' but 'Why am I eating now, and what do I notice as I do so?'

The relevance of this approach is underscored by Irish dietary data across the life course. For example, national surveys consistently report low average fibre intakes among adults and children, despite clear public health recommendations. Fibre-rich foods, such as whole grains, vegetables and legumes, contribute to satiety and help regulate appetite. Yet they are often displaced by refined, less nutrient-dense foods that promote passive overconsumption.

Mindful eating offers a framework for reconnecting eating behaviour with internal physiological signals that may be dulled or overridden in modern food environments. This is particularly important when considering how eating patterns develop and evolve across the life course. It is well acknowledged that early food experiences, family eating practices and social norms play a crucial role in shaping long-term relationships with food. In childhood, external regulation of eating, such as pressure to finish meals or the use of food as reward, can interfere with innate hunger and satiety cues. In adolescence and adulthood, time pressures, stress and social eating often further distance individuals from internal signals.

Importantly, mindful eating must be understood within the broader social and environmental determinants of food choice. Awareness alone cannot overcome structural barriers such as food affordability, availability and marketing practices. However, cultivating awareness of hunger, appetite and eating context can support individuals in navigating these challenges, particularly when combined with public health policies that promote healthier food environments.

This book is written for anyone who senses that something is missing from the way we talk about food. It is for students, practitioners and general readers who want a broader, kinder and more realistic understanding of eating. Grounded in research but attentive to lived experience, it places food back where it belongs. Not just on the plate as a collection of nutrients, but in the rhythms of daily life, in relationships and in the shared culture of eating that has always mattered in Ireland. By grounding mindful eating in national evidence and lived experience, the aim is to move beyond simplistic narratives of 'good' and 'bad' foods and towards a more compassionate, informed and sustainable relationship with eating.

Ultimately, to eat mindfully is not to eat perfectly, but to eat with awareness – of our bodies, our contexts and our cultures. In doing so, we honour food not only as nourishment, but as a central thread in the fabric of Irish life.

DR JANETTE WALTON

PROLOGUE

At twenty-eight years of age, Claudia was diagnosed with a rare intestinal disorder, which causes poor digestion and insufficient uptake of nutrients in the bowel. Multiple surgical interventions and numerous medical treatments did little to help. Doctors at the University Hospital of Zurich decided to treat Claudia with a nutrient solution administered intravenously via a catheter.

Though the nutrient solution contained all the vitamins, essential fats, trace elements, proteins and carbohydrates she needed, Claudia developed symptoms of progressive malnutrition. Her skin lost its colour, she felt exhausted and sluggish, her liver function deteriorated and her body's normal levels of salts and sugars were disrupted. Claudia died at just 31 of a heart attack caused by an excess of sugars in her body. And yet, there was nothing wrong with the dose of sugars in the nutrient solution she had been taking.

I first heard of Claudia's tragic case as a medical student in an internal medicine course. Her story moved me deeply, first and foremost because it was shocking to hear of someone so young dying of a dietary issue, but also because I suffered from gastrointestinal issues myself as a young adult and had to doubt how well my bowel might function. Claudia's death impressed upon me the importance of nutrition in its entirety and it has continued to influence my scientific studies to this day. Even the very latest findings on the science of nutrition cannot explain why she died, because they continue to assume that nutrition is little more than the uptake of nutrients via the blood. According to this school of thought, it doesn't matter whether these nutrients are consumed as tablets, via a catheter, or in an apple. This view continues to be taught as part of medical studies, yet I have observed doctors in hospitals intuitively deviating from it, time and again. Even if a tube-fed solution contains the perfect balance of nutrients, any experienced clinician knows that a patient who eats bread, yoghurt and apple slices in small portions is likely to have a longer, higher-quality life than a patient who is fed artificially.

THE SECRET TO A GOOD, LONG LIFE

People who live to great ages testify to the importance of regularly consuming unadulterated, whole foods. These people typically love traditional foods and live in regions with much-exalted food cultures, such as France, Italy and Japan. A Japanese woman named Kane Takana died in April 2022 at the age of 119, making her the world's oldest woman at the time. Kane always put food and everything connected to it centre-stage.

When war broke out with China in 1937, Kane followed her husband and her son to the front, where she cooked noodles for people in need. After the war, she and her husband converted to Christianity and founded a church. She had felt drawn to Christian culture since childhood, due to the importance of food in Christian spirituality. In 1993, her husband died. At ninety, she developed cataracts, and at 103, she underwent an operation for colon cancer and had to move into a care home. Despite this, she retained her sense of optimism.

In an interview in 2021, beaming from over the bouquet she had received for her birthday, she said, grinning: 'I'm not going to die, the thought hasn't even crossed my mind.'[1] She consciously ate three meals a day of rice, fish and vegetables. She would go for a daily fifteen-minute walk and take part in a quiz once a week. She maintained a sense of good taste to the end. Tea ceremonies and calligraphy exercises helped her to keep her mind sharp and feel connected to a higher reality.

In early 2023, newspapers across the world reported the story of Sister André, who died in her sleep at the age of 118. She lived in southern France and had survived two world wars, the Spanish Flu and a bout of COVID-19. She did not have a devout upbringing but chose to join a religious order to help people in need, spending many years caring for elderly individuals younger than her. She once said she had two primary goals in life: to share her love for the world and not to compromise her own needs. This uncompromising nature revealed itself most clearly in food. She would eat a little chocolate at breakfast and enjoy a glass of red wine at lunch every day. She remained a true gourmet with a complex palate until well into her old age – as evidenced by her penchant for lobster. She celebrated her 117th birthday with a feast of goose liver, roast capon and cheese. Her favourite dessert was baked Alaska, which she enjoyed in small portions: cold ice-cream tucked away under a blanket of hot meringue.

What's remarkable about this story is that Sister André was not the only one. There are plenty of people in France who regularly consume fatty meat and liver, mouldy cheese and sweet desserts and wash it all down with wine. The French are far more reluctant to be influenced by nutritional science and prefer to follow their noses, tongues, eyes and ears. This habit is taught and keenly honed in Mediterranean cultures. Despite this, bon viveurs of this kind tend, on average, to live longer lives and are comparatively less likely to suffer from cardiac issues and cancer. In dietetics, this baffling phenomenon is known as the French Paradox. In France, pleasure – including saturated fatty acids, cholesterol and alcohol – and health can seemingly coexist.

Another concept linked to the French Paradox is the Blue Zones, a term referring to regions of the world where people live to exceptional ages despite the absence of above-average spending on local healthcare systems. They include Sardinia, the Greek island of Icaria, the Japanese island of Okinawa and the Nicoya Peninsula in Costa Rica. The common factor among inhabitants of these zones is that they tend to intuitively eat for pleasure and drink lots of tea and coffee. Yet this pursuit of pleasure is not extravagant; it is closely bound up with traditions and spiritual beliefs. Preserving rituals helps coordinate food consumption and ensures that no one eats more than they need. The idea of deliberately going hungry or counting calories is alien to the inhabitants of the Blue Zones. These are regions where calories are not just consumed, they are savoured in accordance with myths and a sense of deeper meaning.

I wanted to find out more about people who live to great ages, learn more about their unique insights, their feelings and their secrets. To me, Sister André seemed integral to this project; there are dozens of videos in which she discusses her convictions, experiences and life maxims. I discovered that when it came to food, she always trusted her sense of smell and taste, as well as her own intuition. She believed eating was a ritual of great significance. Even in the last year of her life, when she was blind and came to need a wheelchair, she did not tire of emphasising life's great worth and how important it was to share the world's riches, as well as its dishes.

However, while these videos contained plenty of important information, they did little to sate my curiosity; if anything, they piqued it even more. What time did Sister André go to bed? When did she get up? What did she think about snacks between meals? What were her feelings on Brussels sprouts? Was she *regular*?

During this period of curiosity-filled mourning for Sister André, I was visited in the clinic by a French journalist hoping to interview me about my new treatment approaches and to tour the facilities. When the interview was over, I asked if she had ever heard of Sister André. She had, and I was thrilled to hear that she shared my enthusiasm for the 'doyenne de l'humanité', as she is known in France. Yet when I put to her my detailed questions regarding the diets enjoyed by the oldest people alive, she rudely cut me off: 'What does she think about Brussels sprouts? What absolute nonsense. You won't learn Sister André's secret that way. You have to look at it in context.'

Her criticism affected me deeply because I was – I felt – taking a holistic approach. When she saw how disappointed and annoyed I was, she told me a story about her grandmother, Anna, who lived in Germany. She had reached the ripe old age of 103 and remained fighting fit to the end. She was an important figure in the journalist's life, mainly because her father had abandoned the family early on, leaving her mother without a mainstay. Anna always had a very positive attitude; she was an optimist, unflappable. Much like Kane Takana and Sister André, food and the rituals associated with it played a key role in Anna's life. She had experienced starvation in her childhood, so she understood that food was not to be taken for granted, that it was a gift.

Anna had excellent taste and was conscious in her eating habits, enjoying everything in moderation, preferably with fresh ingredients she bought at the market. She didn't drink alcohol due to an allergy. She was always physically active, without ever doing much sport. Her special culinary interest was still mineral water: she kept lots of different types at home because she felt each tasted different and she enjoyed the variety. She knew the telephone numbers of all the water suppliers off by heart well into her old age. She never took dietary supplements, not a single vitamin tablet that her doctor prescribed, because she insisted that everything she consumed be something she could enjoy the taste of on her tongue.

She was modest in all things, including food, but she loved it when doctors praised her body, which was fit as a fiddle even at 100. She loved to tell the story of one trip to the clinic where the doctors and nurses had stood around her bed, marvelling at her immaculate, unblemished legs, or the one about the cardiologist who could hardly believe how young and vigorous her heart was.

The journalist pointed out that her mother and her grandmother had lived in the same house and that, essentially, the same meals were available to both. Their personalities, however, were starkly different. Her mother had not inherited Anna's frugality or her disposition; she belonged to a different generation, one which experienced different things. She had very high expectations of life, which often led to conflict. She laughed at Anna's love of mineral water because, to her, water was just water; lemonade was much nicer. She felt she had the right to eat sweets at any time of day and she would devour the Easter eggs or Christmas pastries she received in a flash. It never would have occurred to Anna to do such a thing. She tended to use these kinds of treats more as decoration and would throw them away afterwards because she liked to decide for herself how she lived and what she ate and didn't want to be tempted by gifts and advertising. By contrast, when the journalist's mother was offered a large glass of wine or a big piece of cake, she would accept without a moment's hesitation. This openness of hers made her likeable, but it also caused significant chaos, suffering and health problems in her own life. Anna was the complete opposite. In her mind, everything was part of a higher order: her background, the dishes she ate, her strict way of eating, her spiritual beliefs – all these things came from within and created a whole.

A serious breakdown in chemical nutrition theory

In early societies, everything to do with food was closely tied to symbolic meanings, magical practices, ceremonies and taboos. This remains the case for traditional societies today, albeit to a lesser extent. It is easy to observe in French food culture. In French, the word *menu* doesn't refer to a choice of dishes but to instructions for how the ritual of a meal ought to proceed. The arrival of fast food, the microwave and increasing time pressure in the workplace saw a waning in the need for every meal to be enjoyed as part of a group ritual, as well as a loss of the slower pace at which such rituals could happen.

At the same time, the false notion began to spread that eating amounts to little more than taking in chemical nutrients, which served as the scientific justification behind the food industry. In addition, fast food would be practically inedible if it were not for the fact that our palates are tricked with vast quantities of added sugar and salt into believing we're biting into something tasty.

In recent times, television, laptops and smartphones have encouraged unconscious eating, where we consume calories joylessly and with abandon. We know what happens when culinary culture backslides to the Age of Reptiles: rates of diabetes have quadrupled since 1980, obesity has doubled, and the number of young people presenting with bowel cancer is rising significantly.[2] With the resounding success of the fast food industry, one in ten people is suffering from an autoimmune disease, most commonly inflammation of the joints, bowel and skin, or arthritis, coeliac disease and allergic skin complaints.[3]

Nutrients such as vitamins and fatty acids are surprisingly lacking in health benefits and may even appear unhealthy when isolated and consumed in tablet form. It is only when understood *in context*, as part of a food framework and embedded within a food matrix, that they reveal their positive effects. Even whole foods are no good on their own; they are always part of a physical and social environment. A dish like Sister André's baked Alaska is much more unhealthy on an empty stomach than after a full meal; the body is not prepared for it, and there is no foundation of salad and vegetables to slow the flow of sugar. Whole foods have to be enjoyed within meals and daily routines for their benefits to shine through. The latest research indicates that breathing and sleep affect how the body absorbs nutrients and regenerates after eating. In the Blue Zones, the social environment and the sharing and spiritual significance of food also influence how healthy a meal is, as several studies have documented.[4] This is also supported by modern sensory physiology, which argues that eating is the most complex and intense form of sensory perception, engaging vast areas of the brain. Eating is also a mental activity and has the potential to expand our consciousness. This is why people who eat mindfully are healthier than those who do not, even if they consume the same nutrients: mindfulness prepares the body for digestion and relaxation prevents unnecessary fat deposits from forming.[5]

Understandably, modern medicine is sorely tempted to ascribe complex health phenomena to mundane chemical processes, despite it becoming increasingly apparent that this strategy is often inadequate for understanding complex systems which are always greater than the sum of their parts. Claudia's death is one poignant testament to this.

In addition, the food industry avoids complexity like the plague because industrial methods are geared toward producing single nutrients cheaply and in large quantities with a long shelf life. Building complex food structures would be much too expensive. Yet the medical, biological and psychological research on this issue increasingly recognises the need to examine food in all its holistic complexity.

It is part of a long tradition. Our relationship to eating and food is a central theme of all spiritual teachings of the last couple of millennia. Eyes see the food. Arms and hands bring it to the mouth. It travels down the oesophagus, through the stomach and into the intestines, where it is digested with the aid of juices produced by the pancreas and the gallbladder. The liver detoxifies whatever has been absorbed so that the nutrients can be distributed throughout the body via the blood. Nutrients are carried to the brain and the sensory organs, to the heart and lungs, the skin and hair, to the abdominal cavity, the sex organs, the bones and muscles and fatty tissue. Several hormones determine how and where substances are transformed and used. Gut bacteria and the immune system are responsible for recognising and removing harmful substances. The kidneys filter out waste products from the blood and excrete them through the bladder. The rectum channels undigested matter out of the body as stool. Nutrients also leave the body via the lymphatic fluid and the skin. It is like a significant current of life, flowing throughout the entire body. Indian scholars called this current 'prana', and it was believed to link the breath, food and higher worlds. Modern biology has confirmed that our bodies possess thousands of receptors in the brain and other organs that capture the flow of nutrients. This provides a scientific explanation for the diverse effects that food exerts on our minds, our social charisma and our consciousness. In practice, this means that when we eat and cook, we can tap into this stream of nutrients, control it, foster it, or disrupt it.

The new science of holistic nutrition

This book aims to demonstrate what can truly nourish us in both body and mind. Each chapter offers practical tips for achieving holistic nutrition. The first chapter examines the observation that people who live to great ages tend to have a markedly good sense of taste and smell, which they continue to hone through mindful eating. What can we learn from them? The second chapter examines the ever-dwindling gap between meal-times and snacks, explaining why this is a problem and what we can do about it. Fasting is the order of the day. In the third chapter, we'll look at healthy foods and why a whole apple is more nutritious than apple juice, despite both being composed of the same chemical molecules. In the fourth chapter, I explore the secrets of eating together and the rituals related to eating that cultures use to establish and maintain social ties. The fifth chapter examines the flow of nutritional energy and provides simple mental techniques to help transform calories into mental, social and spiritual vigour. To stay healthy, the body must rid itself of the remnants of foods that cannot be converted into other substances and so the sixth and final chapter looks at how we can consciously support and guide these cleanup efforts.

Holistic nutritional science expands on the notion of nutrition as a purely chemical phenomenon, incorporating psychological, social, ecological and spiritual elements. The question as to what truly nourishes us begins, of course, with food. The latest research shows that whole foods, which have undergone as little chopping and industrial processing as possible, are the most nourishing. When these foods are eaten together – for example, whole apples, pears and nuts – they have a greater overall nutritional impact. Research into the dining behaviours of people who live to great ages also demonstrates that healthy eating naturally entails a positive attitude to food. Mindful eating, as well as fasting, grants us an intense and direct connection to food, transforming simple units of nutritional value into a psychological experience. Eating together at a table is a good opportunity to integrate this experience into a larger social and spiritual context. Energy circulation begins in the gut, where metabolic processes transfer nutrients to the body. It is a creative process in which new substances and new relationships emerge, for example, via enzymes in gut bacteria. Having run the fiery gauntlet of digestion, nutritional energy must then be transformed into other, subtler energies, such as willpower, kindness and mental agility. Proper nutrition, therefore, always involves extensive energy work, the biological and psychological dimensions of which I hope to explain in detail. Finally, the indigestible components of food must be excreted and the body cleansed, as undigested food remnants can be associated with a range of different illnesses, including Type 2 diabetes, heart conditions, certain cancers and diseases of the brain. What truly nourishes us, then, is not isolated, naked calories but food in its entirety, our attitude to nutrition and the transformation of nutritional energy. I consider this a spiritual approach because it centres on connectedness. It does not simply list a mountain of specialist knowledge; it highlights a specific practice and illuminates a path towards a fulfilled life.

Mindful Eating

Mindful eating is the practice of experiencing food in its entirety. Increasingly, both children and adults eat in front of the television or the computer. Food is eaten so quickly and so inattentively that it is impossible to develop awareness around food and digestion. We remain unaware of the sugar flooding our bodies, or the salt that drives up our blood pressure. By contrast, Kane Takana, Sister André and Grandma Anna concentrated as they ate, doing so consciously to feel what happened in their bodies.

People who eat mindfully retain a good sense of taste and smell, abilities which tend to worsen with age. According to recent research, these senses are vital to long life. One study examined scent perception in 3,000 people aged 57–85, using the scents of roses, leather, fish, oranges and peppermint.[1] People who struggled to identify the scents were four times more likely to die over the next five years than those who could identify them correctly. Other studies also attest to the good sense of taste among people who live to over 100 years of age.[2] The fact that women tend on average to live longer than men, eat more healthily than men and enjoy greater social contact in old age can be tied in significant part to their superior scent perception. Grandma Anna was not joking when she claimed to be able to distinguish between different brands of mineral water by taste; in fact, it was the key to her long life.

Why is our ability to correctly identify scents so important? It helps us tell the difference between polluted and fresh air, distinguish between healthy and unhealthy foods and spot pathogens. It motivates us to eat more nutrient-dense foods, helps us spot hidden calories and salt and ensures we don't consume them unwittingly. But while scent perception is important when choosing our environment and the food we eat, it is also highly significant from a psychological perspective. Pleasant smells lift our mood and provide a feeling of connectedness. Scent perception is also important for living together and anchoring us spiritually within a greater context, as I will demonstrate when we look more closely at the practice of eating together in Chapter Four.

To put it another way: people with a weaker sense of scent perception eat less healthily; they eat a smaller variety of foods, they are less likely to enjoy nature, have fewer social contacts and are less likely to engage with spirituality. In certain circumstances, individuals with diseases of the brain may eat poorly and can suffer from a lower quality of life because the disease restricts their sense of smell.[3] People who do not pick up on sugar eat substantially more of it to get a taste of sweetness, but in doing so, they run the risk of developing Type 2 diabetes. Fortunately, it is possible to train our sense of taste and smell as we would a muscle. We know this because almost all older people can recognise the smell of coffee but not that of roses. This has nothing to do with genetics or changes in the brain; it is simply a matter of circumstance: people tend to smell coffee every day and are less likely to smell roses with the same frequency. Regularly stopping to smell the roses is an effective way of ensuring we can identify roses by scent into old age. However, the practice that matters most for ensuring a long, pleasure-filled life is mindful eating.

Developing mindful eating habits

We ought to plan each day, so we have enough time to eat mindfully. It doesn't take much. A certain degree of relaxation and a proper break from work are necessary prerequisites for mindful meals. Twenty minutes will suffice, but even ten minutes is better than eating while on the phone, at the computer, or on the move. The tragedy of modern culture's distraction is the false notion that the most interesting things are happening outside ourselves. In fact, the most exciting thing of all is happening inside our own bodies.

A good place to start is to look at and smell our food for a few moments, undisturbed. This brings it to the centre of our attention. Sometimes I think about the minerals, the soil, the rain, the plants and the work of numerous people that was required for the food to find its way onto my plate. To develop the habit of mindful eating, we must eat as we usually do while remaining aware that we are eating. When I eat a sandwich mindfully, I think, 'Now I'm eating a sandwich'. It's a little unusual because, usually, when I eat, I don't think about it. I think about my to-do list, or I feel that slight sense of unease when I remember that I still haven't replied to this or that email. My personal motivation for consciously thinking about what I eat is not my health or how I might support it through what I eat; my primary interest is the pleasure I take in it. Eating, even if the meal is dull, is always an immediate, intensely physical experience. This is what makes it so rich in symbolism and so meaningful to human beings. It's why inattentive eating is such a problem. It robs us of the most intense point of contact we have with the world around us. Between bites, I turn my attention time and again to my breathing. It helps to find a rhythm, a midway point between total control and total indulgence. When I'm out with other people, I try to split my attention equally between the food and the people I'm with and really seize the opportunity to talk about the food to deepen my awareness of it.

Mindful eating can almost turn an unhealthy dish into a healthy one, because the quantity and the speed at which we eat make a substantial difference to how nutritious a food is. Even sugar – consumed in small amounts, very slowly and at a relaxed pace – loses its potential to make us ill, because the body can take in each portion and digest it without a spike in blood sugar or an insulin response, with all the consequences that entails.

The opposite of mindful eating is inattentive, stress and emotional eating. When we eat like this, we do not focus on what we are eating; instead, we are consumed by distractions, stress, or complicated feelings. In these situations, we lack control over our food, including its quantity and the speed at which we eat it. This may lead to excessive, joy-free calorie consumption and a disregard for the cues that tell us when we are full. Worse than this, however, is the vicious circle that ensues. Emotional and inattentive eating may lead to noticeable or subconscious feelings of shame and guilt, which, in turn, encourage emotional and inattentive eating.

The advantage of taking pleasure in your food

In my younger days, I spent a few years living and working in the US, where I began eating unhealthily. The US is not a Blue Zone with eating traditions and rituals that have developed over centuries and which serve to protect people against illness and I learned this the hard way. In the second year of my stay, my European eating habits fell by the wayside. I found myself drinking sugary lemonade first thing in the morning, eating sandwiches made with a pound of peanut butter and ultra-sweet grape jam and, in the afternoons, when I felt tired, reaching for a doughnut. I felt ashamed to be eating these kinds of hyper-processed foods – *what would my mother have said?* – and I became increasingly afraid of natural foodstuffs, to the point where I preferred processed rectangular fishfingers to a whole fish. It became a vicious circle in which I numbed my shame and my fear of whole foods by gobbling up calories indiscriminately and to excess. I had bad skin and I gained over ten kilos.

Back in Switzerland, where friends and acquaintances

noticed what poor shape I was in, I found the motivation to end my unhealthy relationship with food. The thing that helped most was eating slowly and mindfully. If I bought myself a doughnut, I'd place a small piece of it in my mouth and fully experience all the sugar and fat spreading across my tongue and then through my body. I observed that I didn't have to eat the whole doughnut to feel good, because this repeated mindfulness practice made even the tiniest pieces of doughnut so thrilling and satisfying that I felt full much more quickly. When it comes to mindful eating, the short-term goal is to eat more slowly and take greater pleasure in eating, so we require fewer calories, less meat and less fast food to feel full and satisfied.

But there's much more to mindfulness than meets the eye. With mindfulness, we can identify and heal psychological processes such as attachments, aversions and illusions as sources of suffering and illness, and cultivate healing mental practices such as thankfulness, humility and kindness. In my case, I noticed that when I was in the US, I fell for the illusion that I needed a doughnut, a sandwich, or both in the afternoon to have enough energy for the rest of the day. Through my mindfulness exercises, I came to feel that the mental connection I was making between sweetness and energy was not benefiting me; it was an attachment, a dependency I needed to rid myself of to feel freer. Step by step, I managed it, and these days I eat nothing in the afternoons. Instead, I go for a walk or do a few gymnastics exercises to boost my energy levels.

Developing intuition around eating

Inattentive eating is a relatively new phenomenon and one that our bodies are not prepared for. Prehistoric individuals had to take great care when sourcing and eating food, not least because many naturally occurring plants are toxic in some form or have no nutritional value for humans. Humans are omnivores, possessing great nutritional intelligence, a powerful sense of taste and smell and a good memory. However, like any other ability, this intelligence and perceptive capacity must be honed. This is why making changes to our diet requires so much effort.

Children and young people who have grown up eating fast foods predominantly composed of maize, soya, wheat and meat, enriched with hidden sugars and salt that mask or mitigate sour or bitter flavours, do not have the opportunity to develop the necessary nutritional intelligence. They must learn how to eat healthily and mindfully, in the same way that you might learn a second language.

Digitisation has the potential to further disrupt nutritional intelligence because our constant media consumption prioritises our senses of sight and hearing – to the detriment of our senses of taste, smell and touch. It is almost impossible to eat mindfully in front of the television because it only serves to bolster the element of distraction, which threatens to overwhelm any possibility of true awareness.

There are profound consequences to this development.

The 1980s witnessed a boom in inattentive eating, leading to an epidemic of obesity, Type 2 diabetes and autoimmune diseases. Nutritional studies demonstrate that one thing in particular can combat the increase in inattentive eating: mindfulness. Diets that tell you *what* to eat but not *how* to eat can only be successful in the short term. Intuitive eating expands upon this, listening to the body's signals to recognise when we are hungry or full, and which tastes we prefer and permitting us to eat in a way that is natural to us, without being led by external rules. Ultimately, mindfulness also involves rules, rituals and intuition, but it complements these elements with a comprehensive process of developing awareness. This permits us to liberate ourselves from attachments to certain foods and the illusions we may have about them. This is particularly important when evaluating the sustainability of a diet.[4]

In Asia, issues such as obesity and overeating are developing at a much more gradual pace because mindfulness plays a greater role in the culture at large and traditional customs act as obstacles to inattentive eating. Confucius felt the use of knives at the dinner table was barbaric. What place did a knife have in a truly mindful relationship with one's food? By contrast, chopsticks allow the diner to enjoy an entirely different, gentler interaction with their food. They can be used to grab food, provided they are used with care. Chopsticks can also be used to separate food without cutting, tearing, piercing or chopping. Chopsticks do not spoil food; instead, they elevate its ingredients and textures.

Ultimately, they act as a support for bringing food to the mouth, rather than acting like a pair of pliers. With chopsticks, food is not prey to be pounced on violently, carelessly; it is transformed, elevated, ready to contribute to a sense of bodily harmony and calm. Of course, Asian culinary customs do not offer absolute protection against inattentive eating. Healthy eating habits are always founded on personal motivation and a nurturing approach.

There is also an ecological element to mindful eating. Eating slowly and mindfully allows us to consider where our food comes from and how it was produced. This can help us choose more organically grown produce. And by eating less, we can afford more expensive, ecologically sound foods. When we eat mindfully, we need less meat, because we appreciate the meat we do eat with greater intensity, meaning smaller portions are better able to satisfy us. Mindful eating can also prompt a deeper connection to nature, raising our awareness of environmental issues and inspiring us to live greener lifestyles.

Spiritual teachers have employed compelling methods to convince their followers of the importance of mindful eating. Jesus, a keen eater and wine drinker, preferred to preach at a table. The night before he went to his death, he broke bread and offered it to his disciples, saying, 'Take and eat, this is my body.' Of course, saying 'Not only is what I'm giving you made from the best ears of wheat and baked with love, but it's also God Himself,' is a fairly extreme call to mindful eating. The

Buddha took a subtler, more effective approach when introducing his monks to mindful eating. He forbade them from earning money to buy food. Consequently, they were entirely dependent on gifts. They would then have to employ mindfulness, using their eyes, ears, fingers, mouths and noses to determine whether the food they received from – often poor – strangers was overcooked, spoiled, contaminated, or edible.

Eating: a full-body experience

Mindful eating is certainly necessary from the perspective of health and morality. Still, it's also an adventure in itself – particularly that first taste, when a food touches the tip of your tongue and then slowly comes into contact with the rest of your mouth. This direct interaction with the outside world warrants closer examination. It is a matter of sensations, a kind of tender desire that affects not only the skin but many other, deeper, softer, more primal parts of the body: the gut and the glands inside it. Food spreads across the vast extent of our mucous membranes, modulating the body's awareness of itself from within and prompting a holistic change in bodily awareness and ultimately consciousness. At its best, it's a feeling of well-being that radiates from every part of the body. Like the mouth, the gut is covered in taste buds and each nerve cell has sensors that detect the flavours of food. It is worth tuning into this full-body event, both critically and simply for the pleasure it brings.

Mindful eating offers an excellent opportunity to

engage all our senses fully. Aside from the five classic senses, we also have a sense of pain, a sense of temperature, a sense of our own bodies, a sense of appetite, a sense of balance, a sense of acceleration and deceleration, a sense of our bodies in space (known as proprioception) and a sense of the passing of time. These enable us to recognise where we are and with whom, what we are eating and how we feel about it.

When we eat, it is important to activate the simplest and most fundamental form of consciousness, namely, bodily awareness. This impacts our awareness and perception of our bodies, including its movements, the positions it takes and the sensations it encounters. It requires countless inner senses that are not among the classic five externally focused senses. It is a matter of sensing our bodies as a whole, interpreting bodily processes and responding to them. Bodily awareness can only be achieved through a combination of internal and external stimuli and internal judgements.[5] Awareness means an openness that allows us to perceive and make best use of a wealth of internal and external information. Imagine you're biting into a strawberry. You mindfully register signals of the strawberry's warmth and softness. You also have a visual impression of the strawberry, you feel the slight crunch as you bite into it and sense its taste and scent. You also notice the position of your body while you're eating, how it changes, the movements in your jaw and all the sensory impressions that arise from the space outside of your body. These are called external or exteroceptive stimuli and as far as the brain is concerned, the mouth belongs at least in part to the external world. Inside the insular cortex, an area on the sides of both hemispheres of the brain, these stimuli are combined with visceral signals from within the body. These internal signals come from the stomach, which is busy processing the chewed-up strawberry; the gut, which digests the strawberry; the heart, which beats a little faster; the breath, which becomes more irregular when we eat; and body temperature, which increases slightly. They primarily reach the brain via the brainstem and have direct access to the limbic system, which is responsible for feelings, emotions, motivation and stress responses. Sensory impressions are then evaluated in the different limbic regions: the amygdala, which supports the insular cortex, determines how much the strawberry corresponds to the person's preferences and the hippocampus compares the strawberry experience to previous, similar food experiences. Since all this can take place without our being conscious of it, it's not uncommon for the body to signal that it is full, that it feels an aversion to a dish, or that it is affected by the unpleasant influence of others at the table before we notice this discomfort ourselves. We may fail to adjust our eating and social behaviour in time.

Bodily awareness also has a significant relationship to the self and how we perceive ourselves. Our original selves, as foetuses and infants, were bodily, i.e. the sense of our active bodies in relation to the bodies of our mothers, to foods, objects and people in our environment.[6] Positive bodily awareness, supported by mindful eating, can lead to a positive self-image and sense of self-esteem. At the same time, mindlessly consuming calories may foster a negative body image, contributing to insecurities and a low sense of self-worth. Furthermore, mindful eating helps us to accept and to value our appetites, our desire for food and our digestion, independent of social norms or ideals. Mindful eating offers a valuable opportunity to develop an authentic feel for one's body. By eating mindfully, we can learn to distinguish between taking pleasure in eating, which stems from the dishes themselves and genuine appetite and social pressure. This allows for a deeper connection with, acceptance of, and love for one's own body and its remarkable abilities. Mindful eating also brings us a sense of self-regulation, a feeling of consciously and thoughtfully listening to our body's hunger and fullness cues, recognising our bodily limits and exerting a positive impact on stress-related appetite, food and gastrointestinal complaints. Mindful eating also helps improve overall emotional resonance, which we need to be in touch with ourselves and our surroundings, and to feel secure and competent in different social situations without isolating ourselves.

Mindful, conscious eating offers the possibility of autonomy and development. Mindfulness is like a space between stimulus and reaction, between seeing a chocolate truffle and eating it. First, the retina captures the truffle's colour, shape and shine. This almost always prompts certain feelings, such as curiosity, anticipation, or shame or guilt. Memories of past experiences with chocolate truffles come to mind. An evaluation then takes place based on these emotions and memories, prompting a mental concept of what it might mean – both emotionally and sensorially – to eat the truffle. The enhanced awareness that mindful eating entails creates space, granting us the power to consciously choose whether to consume a food or to decline it. *Am I addicted to a particular food? Are there other foods that I am repelled by? Why is that? Are the dishes I eat, the way that I eat them and my mindful approach healthy, or harmful?* This delay in our response gives us the freedom and the ability to change.

Mindful eating activates the vagus nerve

It's important to take your time when you eat, for all the reasons listed above. It begins even before you start eating, because your brain needs time to steel your body and your consciousness for ingestion. The hypothalamus, the energy centre, releases a cascade of hormones before eating which prepare our bodies for ingestion. But it pays to be mindful at all stages of eating, not just because ingestion is biologically demanding, but also because it benefits our well-being. Each step can prompt positive feelings: picking up the smell of food at the back of the nose, tasting and chewing it. The intestines, and frankly, the entire body, are full of taste receptors that take pleasure in food. The brain has a special messenger substance, dopamine, which is responsible for rewards. This is released at every stage, continually generating new anticipation.

The whole body is primed to enjoy even the smallest bite – if we give it enough time.

At the same time, the vagus nerve is activated. The vagus nerve connects the brain to the gut, informs the brain of the gut's contents and is one of the body's great parasympathetic nerves. It ensures we stay relaxed so that desire does not turn into greed. The gut and gut bacteria send out fullness signals, which are important for curbing our desire to eat. Fast eaters miss all these different feedback loops, these thrilling conversations between the gut and the brain. They practically eat on autopilot. Our digestive juices, enzymes and bile acids are not adapted to rapid eating. Eating quickly, therefore, leads to indigestion, which can increase the risk of obesity, fatty liver and Type 2 diabetes.

Turning your attention repeatedly to your breath is one of the simplest ways to activate the vagus nerve and increase your awareness. Before I take a first bite of anything, I try to reach a state of calm, focus on my breath and get in touch with my body. As I do this, I ask myself what my needs are in this specific moment and how hungry I actually am. Of course, it doesn't always work and I often forget this exercise altogether due to distractions, lack of attention and stress. But it is worth reminding ourselves repeatedly, because we need oxygen to digest nutrients. Breathing and nutrition are closely linked.

The opposite of pleasurable, mindful eating is eating during which a particular stimulus prompts a chain of addiction-driven, automatic actions. For a time, the bodily self is lost. There is no free will, no autonomy, no person guiding the process, no critical distance between impulse and action. There is now only one site of action. These kinds of binges destroy self-worth in the long term, but even somewhat controlled, if arbitrary, eating habits, perhaps prompted by unthinkingly copying a fashionable diet from some YouTube guru, can alienate us from ourselves, which is why I believe it is unwise to embark on diets uncritically.

For people who have difficulty eating mindfully, keeping a food diary can be helpful. This method is often employed by people suffering from eating disorders or body dissatisfaction, or who have profound feelings of shame around food, prompted by traumatic intimate or food-related experiences. In keeping a diary of this kind, you come to understand how little you know about the type, quantity, colour and quality of the food you have eaten, because we often eat without thinking and without considering what we are eating. Either that, or we eat so quickly that our brains can't keep up with the rapid intake. Conversely, it is a positive sign if you succeed in clearly describing a meal, including the surroundings and the feelings you experienced. Pleasure, after all, requires calm and contemplation. The German language possesses the wonderful word *lauschig*, which can be defined as a kind of pleasant, comfortable state of awareness. Food diaries can help us become more mindful of our eating habits. It can also be beneficial to meditate on our food intake. *Why did I eat? Was it a conscious choice? Did it fit in with my schedule, or was it a spur-of-the-moment decision? Did I eat because I felt genuinely hungry, or were other feelings at play? How did I choose the food? Did I even have a choice? Did I prepare myself to eat with adequate mindfulness and care? Did I eat alone or with others? Did I enjoy the food, or did I consume calories without thinking? How did my feelings of hunger change before and after eating? Why did I stop eating? Was it a conscious decision, or was it simply over?*

Another option is to consciously eat a small dish very mindfully. This is also a method for reducing stress via mindfulness. The Vietnamese monk Thích Nhất Hạnh teaches us to hold a piece of bread in one hand, consider it deeply, and sense that the whole cosmos is contained within it. The earth, sunshine, the farmers, the bakers, all people are contained within this one piece of bread. He then suggests breathing in the scent of the bread to experience the fact that a piece of bread is nothing short of a miracle. Only when we have recognised this and broken out in a happy smile can we then place the piece of bread in our mouths. We are invited to chew the bread and do nothing else. We should not be chewing over our thoughts and worries at the same time. Nhất Hạnh recommends this slow ritual because it can pave the way for mindfulness. Mindfulness can be difficult at first, but it becomes easier with time. The brain and the vagus nerve can be trained. Mindful eating also initiates positive changes in the microbiome, prompting it to develop a more varied language and enabling it to better inform us about our digestion and what our gut needs.

Omnivores like to live dangerously, so they have to be sensitive

Our ancestors were omnivores and nomads, forever exploring new savannahs, forests, coasts and bodies of water. They were repeatedly tasked with appraising new foods. From an evolutionary perspective, it's plausible that our capacity for mindfulness and awareness developed out of this. Just as in very primitive lifeforms, the brain first developed from nerve cells in the lips and mouth, it could also be the case that, in higher animals, self-awareness developed from sensations in the mouth, which is the interface between the internal and the external. The mouth is tasked with determining, both mechanically and chemically, whether to eat something or spit it out, so it has evolved into a sophisticated laboratory capable of assessing poisons and nutrients within seconds. Animals that always eat the same thing do not have a sense of smell or taste. Vampire bats, which feed exclusively on blood, cannot sense sweetness or bitterness, because blood is always of the utmost quality. Carnivores such as cats and dolphins also do not taste their food, because meat is always protein-rich and nourishing. Our openness to the world is revealed in the wide range of foods we eat and this is what made consciousness necessary.

As omnivores, we need tongues sensitive enough to pick out slimy or unusual surfaces and ensure that we don't eat the worm living in the strawberry that we've just popped mindfully between our lips. When we bite into a strawberry, that gentle crunch means it's fresh. If there's no sound and no resistance, it's a sign that the strawberry is too soft, potentially spoiled and should be spat out. If we've taken a first bite and no alarms have been raised, the sensors activate, gauging and intensifying the strawberry's taste. Our expectations – presumably of eating a delicious strawberry – play a key role in this. Saliva partially breaks down and digests the strawberry, allowing more flavours to be released and enhancing flavour perception. If the strawberry tastes surprisingly bitter, we will spit it out, because bitterness can indicate the presence of toxins. Snakes have long tongues, which enable them to clarify all this information before they swallow a bite – a perfectly reasonable course of action when it comes to avoiding poisoning. We ought to be more understanding when children try a new meal by sticking out their tongues.

Our sense of taste determines what flavours are dissolved in the fluid in our mouths. It does this by reducing millions of possible flavours down to just a few fundamental qualities: sweet, salty, bitter, sour and umami. Our mouths also have sensors which detect wateriness, fat content, warming or cooling effects and spiciness. We can include these under the umbrella of our sense of taste, which is primarily aimed at assessing the safety and nutrient content of every bite.

Our sense of smell detects flavours in liquids and in the air. It has hundreds of sensors at its disposal, ideally suited to identifying a wide range of possible flavours. It detects the presence of individual flavours, as well as combinations typical of humans, animals and plants. This is, of course, handy for eating, but it can also help estimate a person's stress levels, identify illnesses and foster a sense of well-being in a familiar home. People with a poor sense of smell generally have fewer close friends, less sex and less zest for life.[7] Social consequences such as these were confirmed during the COVID-19 pandemic, when anosmia temporarily became a common complaint. Poor scent perception is also a cause of accidents, infections, food poisoning and fires, because people with poor scent perception cannot detect the unpleasant scents of smoke, spoiled food, harmful bitter substances and pathogens.

The senses of smell and taste work together closely; what is particularly remarkable about this is that information relating to taste reaches the brain stem 'from below' and olfactory information flows directly into the cerebral cortex and the limbic emotional centre via the olfactory bulb via the nose, i.e. 'from above'. The result of these amazingly complex flows of information, which involve the whole brain, is known as flavour perception. New flavour receptors continue to be discovered across the entire body, be they in the gut, pancreas, or sex organs. And the brain doesn't just receive flavour information from the nose and mouth; every individual nerve cell in the brain has sensors for tasting flavour substances in the blood. One of these flavours is ammonia, which is present in our stool and it smells pretty terrible as far as our noses are concerned. Yet the taste sensors in our gut have no fear when it comes to ammonia; in fact, they're almost drawn to it. Deep inside our intestines, something has an appetite for toilet-related smells, because they indicate that we have eaten well.[8]

What a mess: industrially processed food

Industrially processed food is a relatively new and serious challenge to our sense of flavour, and it represents another threat to mindful eating, alongside smart-phones, television, computers and radio. The food industry enhances its products with cheap, super-stimulating flavours to create a brief, intense and addictive flavour experience. All this feeds into the billions of dollars in profits and increases the influence of food manufacturers, but is ultimately paid for by consumers, potentially leading to a long-term reduction in both pleasure and health. These super-flavours include high quantities of sugar, salt, glutamate and cheap fats.

Industrial ultra-processing can also disrupt the food matrix – the physical structure of a food, such as cell walls and muscle fibres – reducing flavour perception, increasing appetite, blunting our sense of flavour, accelerating the uptake of nutrients, inhibiting feelings of fullness and massively restricting our ability to identify good, varied foods from among monotonous, poor ones. Fibres are crushed, such that it is no longer possible to discern whether a food has aged (typically determined by observing broken fibres). All this leads to macronutrients such as carbohydrates and fats being consumed in quantities that may contribute to overweight and obesity. The industry also sterilises foods, eschewing long molecules in favour of short ones that can be digested quickly. However, overprocessed foods of this kind only nourish the upper part of our gut, totally disregarding the mucous membranes and microbiome in the lower section and in the large intestine.

A whole host of studies demonstrate that adding essential nutrients, which the industry can produce cheaply and in large quantities (such as vitamins and omega-3 fatty acids), may not solve the problem and, when combined with high-dose supplement use, can provide too much of specific nutrients for these users.[9] Industrially produced foods can lack a diverse array of nutrients, an intact food matrix, and the abundance of micronutrients and probiotics found naturally in plants and fungi. Evolution has shaped our tastes so that we instinctively seek out high-energy foods that are naturally rich in micronutrients, structural substances, and fibre. Still, the food industry has made it impossible for us to rely on our perceptual faculties anymore. We have to consciously select foods and retrain our sense of flavour to face this new challenge.

Sweet heaven and hell

Milk and honey are both foods that nature produces for the sole purpose of nourishing living beings. Interestingly, these natural foods are both fairly sweet. Our weakness for sweet things is so great that even hunter-gatherer peoples such as the Hadza prefer a few spoons of honey to a whole piece of meat, despite meat proteins being more vital for body composition.

Human beings view sweetened foods as a kind of cure-all. They can suppress pain and a wide range of unpleasant sensations and memories.[10] They can also provide a sense of security, connection, belonging and even love. Heart-shaped treats on Valentine's, wedding and birthday cakes, Lebkuchen and baked foods at Christmas – these are all testament to the soothing power of sweetness. Any disruption to our sense of flavour – following chemotherapy, for example – typically sparks a preference for very sweet dishes, because sweet flavours provide security amid a cacophony of flavours.[11]

It is probably why all religions and spiritual traditions connect sweet flavours with deities, ancestors, or a higher world. In Islam, Muslims break their Ramadan fast with sweet dates. In the Bible, God promises his people a land flowing with milk and honey. God saves his people in the desert by providing them with sweet manna from heaven. Jesus gives humanity his body, the Bread of Life. In Psalms, sweetness is akin to experiencing God directly: 'Taste ye and see, for the Lord is sweet; blessed is the man that hopeth in him.' Medieval mystics expanded on this understanding of God. The spiritual eroticism of the German mystic Mechthild von Magdeburg is particularly striking: 'I am hoarse in the throat of my chastity, but the sugar of Thy sweet gentleness has made my throat sound once more, that I may sing: Lord, Thy blood and mine are one, unspoiled. Thy love and mine are one, inseparable.

Thy gown and mine are one, immaculate. Thy mouth and mine are one, unkissed by any man but Thee alone.'[12]

In Freud's psychoanalysis, the mild sweetness offered at the mother's breast acts as the infant's bridge to basic trust in the mother and in the world. Lactose is less sweet than sucrose and fructose, probably to ensure that a baby does not develop undue dependency on its mother. When the image of God or the mother figure as sweetness came into being, no one could have foreseen that, one day, every sip and every bite would taste intensely sweet thanks to the addition of refined sugar. In the Bible, God hid among the clouds before appearing unexpectedly as manna. Like the manna, he disappeared again without any apparent reason, only to reappear later on mountains or in rainbows. So it was with sugar, its sweetness suddenly delighting the human consciousness, with the discovery of ripe fruits, or honey, or at the Last Supper. At the beginning of the modern era, a different image of God came to the fore: one who was all-present, all-seeing and all-powerful.

In parallel, sugar began to be produced in ever greater quantities thanks to the labour of enslaved individuals on vast plantations in America and the Caribbean. It would soon become a powerful nutrient, the one we are familiar with in abundance today and which finds its way into salad dressings, ketchup, mayonnaise, pasta sauce, sandwich spread, gherkins, pickled herring, sausages, pickled cabbage, yoghurt, muesli, cereal bars, iced tea, lemonade and bitter schnapps. If trust in artificial foods is to be sustained, the soothing effects of sugar must be present in every bite. 'Don't worry,' it says, 'You can trust what you're eating, it's good.'

Unfortunately, this isn't true. Yes, sugar is an essential fuel for our bodies, but consuming sugar in forms that rarely occur naturally creates oxidative stress, which damages cells and can lead to various illnesses such as heart problems, cancer and diseases of the brain.[13]

There's also the risk of glycation, in which sugar reacts with the walls of the blood vessels and causes them to harden. Glycation is a similar chemical process to one you can observe at home when toasting a slice of bread: the sugars in the bread bind together with proteins in the bread to create a hard, dark crust. But while this makes toast delicious, it's not such good news for our blood vessels. In fact, it stimulates a harmful ageing process that hardens and rigidifies blood vessels, raising blood pressure and overloading the heart.

Sugar also causes the body to release excess insulin, leading to an insulin spike. Insulin increases feelings of hunger, makes us feel tired and signals our bodies to store fat. For all these reasons, our blood must contain only minimal amounts of sugar, i.e. no more than a gram per litre. This is so low that when we have a nosebleed or a cut inside our mouths, our blood tastes salty, bitter, or metallic, rather than sweet.

These medical facts may seem somewhat depressing at first glance, but there is cause for optimism. By avoiding sugar spikes through mindful eating, consuming low-sugar foods and fasting, it is possible to mitigate and sometimes prevent the conditions described above, as well as mitigate depression, migraines, heart problems and even cancer.[14]

Mindful, slow eating is one of the most effective immediate actions we can take, because our bodies are capable of processing dietary sugars healthily to a certain extent and the extent to which they can is determined by the quantity of sugars consumed per minute. The more slowly we eat, and the less we eat, the healthier our food is, even if what we're eating is fast food or a chocolate cake. In another case for optimism, it would be possible to save billions in healthcare costs and prevent a great degree of suffering by introducing laws to limit the sugar content in processed foods, without restricting the pleasure we take in eating them, because our ability to consciously pick up on the amount of sugar we are eating is astonishingly unreliable. For example, in England, a bottle of Fanta contains approximately 15 grams of sugar. In Germany, it contains about 30 grams, whereas in India, Vietnam and Ecuador, it contains about 40 grams. Despite this, there have been no known instances of tourists in England complaining about the poor quality of the local Fanta.

Mindful eating is key to resisting the aggressive, mighty Sugar God, helping us rediscover the finer, mellower natural sweetness of the much older, elemental Sugar Goddess. Ultimately, the sugar used in processed foods is just one source of sweetness among many. In the Blue Zones, where locals take pleasure in food and live to great ages, every dish begins with chopping an onion and some celery, which develops a wonderful sweetness when gently fried. You can smell the sweetness, which lends dishes stability and a kind of trustworthiness without containing too many harmful sugars. Traditional and home-cooked dishes typically contain significantly less sugar than ready-made products and modern restaurant food.

Fruit teas are a good way to rediscover natural sweetness mindfully. When enjoyed mindfully, fruit teas reveal a surprisingly intense sweet taste, despite containing few sugar molecules. Fruit teas are produced by chopping fruits into small pieces and drying them, a practice which can easily be carried out at home. In Germany, hibiscus flower and rosehip blends are particularly popular. Cinnamon is a natural way to sweeten tea. Similarly, rooibos offers our taste buds a gentle sweetness and a slight nutty flavour, while containing a small amount of sugar that our bodies can easily digest. When steeped for longer, red tea is rich and full-bodied and you need only breathe in its warm and woody notes to feel the benefits. Rooibos is also thought to be good for the liver, helping to detoxify it after a sugar shock. Oolong tea is a blend of black and green tea, perfect for honing your ability to appreciate subtle sweetness. Tea is generally well-suited for consumption alongside food. You can drink a small amount before eating to cleanse your mouth and sharpen your taste buds. However, liquids dilute our digestive juices, so it's best to consume larger quantities alongside or after a meal. This enables the body to convert the food into nutrients that can be absorbed.

But you don't have to be a tea lover to enjoy an audience with the gentle Sugar Goddess. Most foods – particularly bread, pasta, potatoes and rice – contain high quantities of carbohydrates. Chewing these types of carbohydrates slowly, thoroughly and mindfully reveals just how sweet they are, such that you'll be unlikely to need added sugars in the form of sauces or ketchup. However, if you can't taste the sweetness in fruit teas at all, you might be suffering from a serious case of blunted taste buds, which significantly increases the risk of being overweight and developing diabetes. If so, it's time to find alternative strategies to combat the saccharification process in foods.

Artificial sugars can offer support with this. They are like angels, lacking the sacred and soul-stirring impact of pure sugar and instead hinting at and representing the fearsome Sugar God himself, without wreaking havoc on our blood vessels. I recommend undertaking a little experiment to get to know these artificial sugars better and see how they compare. In a blind taste test, I easily distinguished between real sugar and artificial sweeteners. Xylitol, which comes from birch bark, is most like sugar in terms of its fullness and heart-warming properties, followed by erythritol, which occurs naturally in small amounts in honey and melons, but is less rounded and less sweet and also contains fewer calories. Stevia, which purports to be the healthiest sweetener available, comes from the tropical Stevia plant and contains almost no calories. It is characterised by a liquorice-like flavour and a faintly bitter aftertaste. Unfortunately, the latter has led to limited success as a sweetener in fast food and soft drinks. 'Zero sugar' foods generally contain a blend of different sweeteners. Green Cola was an exception to this rule, containing only Stevia and it was probably the healthiest cola ever to be on the market. Unfortunately, sales numbers were disappointing and the drink was pulled in most countries.

Other sugar alternatives include cyclamate and saccharin, as well as a combination of the two, known as Assugrin. They are cheap and popular, but can have a metallic, bitter aftertaste in their pure form. None of these sweeteners is particularly healthy, but they may be more nutritious than sugar itself. This remains the case despite the occasional news story claiming that large quantities of saccharin cause cancer and can change the microbiome. Still, we do not ingest the necessary amounts to cause these kinds of side effects.[15] However, high sugar intake has also been associated with dysbiosis (an imbalance of gut bacteria) and other diseases, including those related to dental health. Artificial sweeteners have a more bitter taste and are less addictive than sugar, leading to less attachment to the product than sugar might. This also means that the path from artificially sweetened teas to fruit teas is shorter than the path from sugary teas to fruit teas. Artificial sweeteners are in no way perfect – from a health and taste perspective – but they offer significant support in moving away from sugar.

I will finish with a few words on the sugar rush phenomenon. A sugar rush is unique to real sugar and makes us feel as if we suddenly have more mental energy. Unfortunately for us, it does no such thing. A sugar rush occurs within the dopamine system – the same place stimulated by cocaine – and very briefly boosts concentration and willpower. However, this effect has nothing to do with the nutritional energy sugar provides. A sugar rush takes effect within a few minutes, while its metabolic effects do not occur until half an hour later. Similarly, we now know that sugar prompts a spike in insulin, which makes us hungry and tired – the opposite of what we were hoping for. What's more, consumers of sugar-sweetened beverages experience a rush within seconds, and no substance is capable of travelling from the mouth to the brain at such speeds, meaning that it's a simple case of anticipation combined with the placebo effect. In fact, studies confirm that energy drinks do precisely the opposite of what they claim: they cause tiredness and reduced alertness.[16] All this makes the case for taking a more critical approach to sugar rushes and the advertising that accompanies them.

In conclusion, a mindful sense of sweetness can help us avoid foods that contain too much sugar and enjoy them more slowly. In the long term, we must find ways to eat and drink mindfully, allowing ourselves to discover not merely the Sugar Goddess but the holy power and love in every flavour – including umami, bitterness, sourness and salt. The following passages hope to do just that.

The Magic of Umami

People in the world's Blue Zones enjoy food to the fullest without over-sweetening it, and they were doing so long before artificial sweeteners were discovered. Alongside mindful eating and dining rituals, one factor has proven key to solving this puzzle. In 1909, the Japanese scientist Kikunae Ikeda discovered a fifth taste, which he named 'umami'. The Japanese 'umai' means 'tasty' and 'mi' means 'taste'. In my native German, 'umami' has been translated as 'hearty', 'delicious', 'aromatic', 'earthy' and 'meaty' and I must take umbrage at the latter. Umami has very little to do with meat; in fact, carnivores do not have a sense of umami. Herbivores developed an understanding of umami to identify proteins in plants.[17] We can conclude from this evolutionary story that the sense of umami plays a key role in orienting our nutrition towards plant products, which benefits both our health and the planet. When it comes to mindful eating, our perception of umami needs to last longer – unlike how we experience refined sugars. This offers a critical benefit in terms of mindful, slow eating and calorie reduction. When we eat soup with high umami content, its intense, delicious flavour prompts us to eat less and more slowly, which benefits our health.

Umami is stimulated by components of proteins, among them the amino acid glutamate. Combinations of tomatoes, mushrooms, cheese – especially Parmesan – anchovies, salami, air-cured ham and bacon, all of which contain a high proportion of protein, stimulate our sense of umami to the max. Alongside these more natural flavours, there are also artificial umami flavours. Large quantities of pure glutamate are commonly used in fast food and seasonings, typically as monosodium glutamate (MSG). However, pure glutamate is neither particularly pleasant nor enjoyable; in fact, it's a bit bland and slightly soapy. It's why such large quantities of glutamate are required to give dishes that umami flavour, which is not a healthy practice. By contrast, traditional foods only need a small quantity of glutamate to enhance the flavour, because other protein components, such as ribonucleotides, intensify the glutamate's umami flavour. Spaghetti with tomato sauce and parmesan, or a pizza with tomatoes, cheese and salami, contains natural glutamate in a perfect blend of proteins. It's no coincidence that these dishes, loved the world over, are veritable explosions of i.

Buddhist monks created soups with ample umami to make vegetarian cooking more appetising. In doing so, they discovered that dried mushrooms and tomatoes provide a stronger umami hit than fresh ones. They also found that the darker the mushroom, the more umami flavour it contained, which is why shiitake, morels and porcini are particularly prized for their flavour-enhancing abilities. These ingredients aren't obligatory, however. Most soup recipes serve as a guide for creating umami flavours, as cooking releases the umami compounds in plant proteins. Gently stewing or cooking meat for a long time also helps draw out umami flavours from animal proteins. Stewed for hours over a low flame, a cooking pot filled with oxtail or an ossobuco with minced beef, vegetables and tomatoes becomes a festival of umami flavours. In French, the word *ragoûter* means 'to tantalise the palate' and this is precisely what umami achieves after long hours of cooking. Umami not only transforms the taste of a dish but also makes soups and sauces feel thicker and more nourishing on the tongue. Umami makes the diner feel that there are more nutrients and calories in each mouthful than there are, and this is a good method of weight control, providing you eat mindfully and are conscious of your body's fullness cues.

Another benefit of umami flavours is their ability to make unpleasant-tasting dishes more palatable. Even small portions of calf, chicken, and fish liver contain large quantities of important nutrients, including folic acid, riboflavin, vitamin B12, and thousands of others that we don't even know about yet. From a health perspective, it makes sense to eat a portion of liver once a month, but unfortunately, many people do not enjoy liver due to its bitter flavour. Soaking liver in water or milk can help reduce its bitterness, and the umami in tomatoes, mushrooms and anchovies can further reduce it. The same applies to bitter vegetables, famously loathed by children. Umami can also help boost a desire for protein-rich foods in old age and in people with certain diseases of the brain.

All in all, the magic of umami boasts enormous potential for us, our health and our environment by making it easier to eat fewer calories and less meat without compromising on pleasure.

Salt: a connection to the source

When a child suckles at its mother's breast, it not only experiences the magical sugar and umami flavours of breast milk, it also tastes its mother herself, her sweat and, thus, the substance that is at the foundation of all life: salt. People and animals are mainly composed of salt water and all the fluids we secrete are salty. Salt regulates water content in body tissues, facilitating the transmission of signals to neurons, muscle contractions and helping neutralise strong acids. The great physiological importance of salt stems from our origins in the oceans, where life developed in salt water. It explains why we can forego sugar and umami flavour enhancers altogether, but not our regular intake of salt.

The need to remember our origins in the oceans through consuming salt has led salt to acquire spiritual significance across cultures. In the Indian tradition, the great sages used the image of the sea to illustrate for their students that Atman, the self and Brahman, the cosmos, were identical. They explained that we couldn't distinguish between the taste of salt on our skin, in our sweat and our sexual secretions and the saltiness of the sea, bringing into focus the pantheist teaching that God is in everything. Fittingly, the Indian sages referred to the sense of the interconnectedness of everything as 'oceanic'. When the Buddha emphasised that his teachings had only one flavour – that of salt – he was underscoring their simplicity and elemental quality. In doing so, he also picked up the much older Indian thread of oceanic feeling: the parity of the internal and the external, of the macrocosm and the microcosm, on which his teachings are founded. The American psychologist William James also used the image of the ocean to express the kinship and connection between our souls: 'We are like islands in the sea, separate on the surface but connected in the deep.'[18]

However, while salt is vital for life, a daily salt intake of over two grams can raise blood pressure, which – alongside glycation caused by sugar – is the second most significant cause of stiffening in the blood vessels. Salt consumption has risen sharply since the introduction of processed foods and currently stands at 3.5 grams per day, almost twice the suggested amount. This explains why reducing salt intake to 0.5 grams per day is as effective as blood pressure medication for lowering blood pressure.[19] Savouring salt mindfully allows us to use less of it, which contributes significantly to keeping blood vessels supple and flexible in the long term.

Despite these findings, almost every professional cooking class begins with a call for 'More salt!' because under-salting is the most common reason given for an unsatisfactory dish. This flies in the face of what my grandfather taught me: 'Be careful with the salt, you can always add it in, but you can never take it out!' Salt can turn food into nibbles, soften cucumbers, take the bitterness out of aubergines and lend gin a savoury flavour reminiscent of the sea. If you want to keep salt intake low, it's best to add it early in the cooking process and sprinkle it from a height to ensure it dissolves and is well distributed throughout the dish. Salting at the table requires significantly more salt to achieve the same level of salinity.

Unlike good cooks, who use a little salt to significant effect, the processed food industry employs a raft of chemical tricks to sneak unhealthy quantities of salt into dishes unnoticed, such as adding certain fats and refined sugars. The aim is to lead consumers to believe that the dish is fresher and more nutritious than it really is. It's so successful, in fact, that salt is the second most frequently used additive in processed foods after sugar. Tinned peas, for example, can contain one hundred times more salt than peas from your garden. Marketing strategists have also succeeded in twisting information in medical textbooks, touting the idea that we need isotonic or mineral-enriched drinks for optimal fitness, with a salt content that matches the salt content of our own bodies. This strategy has also prevailed because the increase in blood pressure prompted by consuming salt gives us a temporary feeling of strength and power. However, isotonic and salt-enriched drinks can strain the kidneys and blood vessels, lowering overall fitness in the long term and potentially reducing our lifespan.[20]

The sourness of change

One of the important functions of salt is neutralising acids in our bodily fluids. Just as we have our origins in the sea to thank for our love of salt, our aversion to acids and sour foods is similarly a legacy of our long prehistory in the depths of the oceans, where acid can impair breathing and oxygen uptake. Unlike sweet, salty and umami, which give us a sense of security, sour and bitter flavours signal danger. But this rating system is a little outdated. In the age of industrial processing, salt and sugar have become threats to our health, while sour and bitter foods, such as fruit, vegetables and fermented foods, are among the healthiest. Acid is also a sign that healthy, live bacteria (probiotica) are present. Furthermore, plant-based foods are more likely to be bitter and sour, and we can only take in the quantity of plant-based foods our health, our planet and our fellow animals need if we learn to approach sour and bitter flavours without fear and misgivings. In my view, we will not be able to avoid using mindful eating to reconsider our instincts and adapt to our circumstances as they are today. The following passages on acid are intended to encourage and foster this process.

First, a few words on the chemistry of acids. Acids are substances with the capacity to transfer hydrogen ions, also known as protons, to other substances. The opposites of acids are bases, also known as alkalis, which can take on hydrogen ions. The body's balance of hydrogen ions must be precisely calibrated because it significantly affects all biological processes, including cell growth, cell structure, metabolism, muscle movement, nerve conduction and brain function. This adjustment is also known as the acid-base balance and its job is to keep the quantity of free hydrogen ions constant. Imagine it like a game with a precise number of balls. If there are too many or too few balls in circulation, it's impossible to play the game. The pH level indicates the excess of acid; the scale numbers from 0 to 14. Confusingly, a low number means that a solution is acidic, or that there are many balls in play, while a higher number indicates a surplus of alkali, or fewer balls. A pH of 7 indicates a balance of acid and alkali. All our bodies' tissues have an ideal pH level: our blood and brains are neutral, our skin, stomachs and vaginas are acidic, our livers and guts are basic and our urine is the great equaliser, adjusting to the needs of our metabolism.[21]

Our metabolism constantly produces large amounts of acids and bases. Consider stomach acid, which, with a pH of 1, contains ten times more acid than vinegar, which has a pH of 2. The body is constantly producing and disposing of this heavy-duty acid. It has several biological systems for identifying a slight drop in, or excess of, acids in any area of tissue and immediately balancing it out. This speedy chemical balancing act is known as buffering. The blood and much of the body's tissue serve as acid buffers and the lungs are similarly capable of removing excess carbon dioxide, thereby reducing the number of balls in play within minutes. Eventually, however, excess acid produced by metabolism and by eating must be excreted via the urine. The notion that our bodies must constantly fight to prevent overacidification can cause real anxiety, mainly as an excess of acid characterises many healthy foods, or, to put it another way, they contain a significant number of balls that it's someone's job to catch. Lemon juice and vinegar both have a pH of 2, making them the most acidic foods found in the kitchen, followed by orange juice (pH 3) and fermented foods and drinks such as yoghurt, coffee, wine and beer (pH 4). Even milk and honey, both natural foodstuffs, are relatively acidic, with pH values ranging from 4 to 6.5. Human breastmilk is also acidic. In fact, we rarely eat alkaline foods. The main exceptions to this rule are egg white and baking powder, both of which have a pH of 8.

The pH levels we perceive as sour tastes in our mouths do not precisely correspond to the body's actual acid load; bases produced during digestion balance out the acids. The quantities of acid we take in are generally vanishingly small compared to the acids produced by our metabolism. Just as a fly landing on your shoulder is unlikely to cause a backache, acids in foods do not present any real challenge to the body's acid-base balance.[22] Our bodies could neutralise a litre of vinegar in a heartbeat.

Now let's turn to enjoying acids mindfully. Our tongues are amazing natural pH-measuring devices, constantly monitoring numbers of hydrogen ions and passing that number on to the brain, which in turn transforms that chemical acid into a sensation of sourness and, occasionally, a shift in consciousness. This chapter aims to explain how we can enjoy this feeling without the anxiety that sometimes accompanies it. And this is where fermentation comes into play. Fermentation is a natural process in which microorganisms (such as bacteria, yeasts, or moulds) convert sugars and starches in foodstuffs into acids. This process extends the shelf life of foods, promotes healthy digestion, increases their nutritional content and makes them crunchy and fresh-tasting.

Human beings are not the first in the animal kingdom to discover the significant benefits of fermentation. Squirrels bury acorns to allow them to go sour and some bird species have a crop where seeds ferment, making them easier to digest. Compared to most other animals, however, humans do appear to be particularly keen on sour flavours. To some extent, we have already overcome our primal fear of acidic foods. Fermentation has become one of our key methods for cooking without heat. We need only look at the overwhelming cultural significance and health benefits of sourdough, sauerkraut and even wine and beer. When we eat acidic foods, dopamine in the brain's reward system responds by paying out a premium, which we experience as a sour kick. Despite this, almost all children have an aversion to sour foods, which is why huge quantities of unhealthy sugar often mask the sour flavours in fermented foods like children's yoghurts.

Biting into a sour apple is a real challenge for people who don't experience any significant kind of sour kick, and it's a reaction that must be overcome not just once but at practically every meal, because a third of our foods are fermented. It is believed that around 5000 years ago, people in the Middle East discovered that milk turns sour and coagulates when exposed to sunlight and warmer temperatures. This probably did not provoke much interest at first – at least no more than when you go to add milk to your coffee or pour it over your muesli and find it has turned lumpy and sour. Fortunately, however, some bright spark eventually discovered there was no need to throw away coagulated milk. Instead, it could be salted and turned into a tasty, less perishable foodstuff, such as kefir or yoghurt. In fermentation, salt and acid work closely together. When making sauerkraut, the amount of salt added is crucial to ensuring that the beneficial, acid-forming lactobacilli thrive and can assert themselves over other bacteria. It also determines the fermentation rate, which affects the flavour and crunchiness of the final product.

In small amounts, salt and acidity can enhance each other's perception on the tongue. For example, a little salt added to gin, which is very sour with a pH of 4, can intensify its flavours, creating a tastier drink. When you prepare to take a shot of tequila (pH 3) by putting salt on your tongue, the salt softens the acidity of the spirit.[23] Conversely, it also means we are less able to detect the salt in more sour foods, such as kiwis. It is important to add only a little salt to sour foods, because we can't taste it and our natural sense of how much salt is too much fails to kick in.

Sugar and acid are also closely connected. While acid provokes anxiety, sugar calms us down (though, unfortunately, this comes with several adverse side effects). Even plants have learned that animals exhibit an exaggerated fear of acids, which is why they fill their sour fruits with plenty of sugar, so that animals are motivated to gobble them up and spread the seeds. The processed food industry has taken a leaf out of nature's book. It adds large quantities of sugar to lemonade, vinegary ketchup and salad dressings to mitigate the sour, fresh flavour. It's a shame because acids reduce the rate at which insulin is released and smooth out sugar spikes, doing our blood vessels a world of good in the process. This effect is turned on its head for sweetened products, which stimulate the insulin system. The calming effects of acid are no match for a tsunami of sugar.

Embracing naturally fermented foods

Mindful eating helps us to learn to appreciate acids and eat less sugar as a result. Overcoming a fear of acidic foods essentially entails a form of exposure therapy: coming face to face with something over and over until you ultimately adjust to it. It works very well for acids. Somehow, our genetic programming already understands that the oceanic fear of acids we carry today is overblown – otherwise it would never have created the sour-kick reward system. Exposure is easy. Pick up some naturally sour foods such as fresh alpine clover, rhubarb, sorrel, or apple cider vinegar and every day you can take the next step on your mindful journey through a land of sour delights. Instead of buying a sugar-filled salad dressing at the supermarket, make your own vinaigrette from oil, vinegar, salt and pepper. Natural yoghurt is another great sour snack. If it's too sour for you, sweeten it with a little jam and observe how the sugar softens the sour flavour. The latter has the advantage of letting you decide for yourself how much sugar to add. As your love of sour foods grows, you can continue to reduce the amount of jam you use.

Fermentation is a good strategy for tackling a fear of acidic foods because acids you produce yourself can prompt less anxiety than unfamiliar ones. Making your own sauerkraut can be a good entry point into fermentation and developing a confident relationship with acidic foods. It's easy, too. Just recently, I set out to introduce my children to the miracle of lacto fermentation. I shredded a cabbage before tipping it into a bowl. It weighed exactly one kilo, so I added fifteen grams of salt to the cabbage and kneaded it in for ten minutes. I then poured the cabbage and the liquid it had produced into a pickling jar, packed it tightly and weighed it down with ceramic stones (if there is not enough cabbage water to cover the cabbage, you can always add a little tap water). After that, I left the cabbage to ferment at room temperature in the shade for a month, stirring it daily and making sure to pack it tightly and keep it below the water level. The process enabled us to hear, smell and see fermentation in action, and to witness the transformative power of lactic acid bacteria up close. Initially, my children hated the smell of fermenting cabbage, comparing it to a never-ending fart. They were reassured to learn, however, that this is normal and that the scent comes from enterococci – gut bacteria – which are replaced by more appetising lactic acid bacteria over the course of the fermentation process.

After four days, I put the jar in the cellar, where the cooler temperature would benefit the lactic acid bacteria. After four weeks, my children confirmed that the fart smell had disappeared entirely and the cabbage was wonderfully crunchy and sour. Unfortunately, they still didn't like the taste, but at least I was able to take them on a little culinary voyage for those few weeks. Included in these trips was a treatment with top-quality healthy bacteria. A gramme of sauerkraut contains between ten million and one billion live probiotics. Unlike the many probiotic products available at the chemist's – which include a smaller quantity of probiotics – the quantity present in homemade sauerkraut is significant enough that a sizeable number of bacteria will survive the acidity of the stomach and make their way into the gut. Even shop-bought sauerkraut does not have the same effect because, like almost all fermented products, it is pasteurised, destroying the probiotics.

I decided to follow up my mindful journey into the land of sauerkraut with another experiment. This time, I opted for kimchi, its sourness enhanced with bitter and spicy flavours. The first kimchi I ever tried was from a supermarket and I found it bland and disappointing. There was a monotonous acidity and the cabbage was completely limp. Fortunately, I didn't stop there; I tried again with some kimchi from the farmers' market, made by a Korean woman according to her mother's recipe. It was pretty expensive, but my investment paid off. The cabbage was crunchy with a tantalising, sour flavour with subtle fruity and bitter notes. It left a refreshing sensation on my tongue and in my throat, which lingered pleasantly for a whole hour. It served to cement and reinvigorate my love of sour foods.

Kefir is another fermented foodstuff. It is very popular in the Middle East, the birthplace of fermentation. Even the Prophet Muhammad, who worked as a shepherd in his younger years, is said to have enjoyed kefir and heartily recommended it. It's exceedingly easy to make. Kefir grains consist of various bacteria and yeasts and you can buy them in the shops or online. Stir them into a litre of whole milk, leave to stand in a warm room for thirty-six hours, then place in the fridge for twelve hours to cool and hey presto, you've got kefir. I made some kefir while working on this passage and it was so sour that it certainly gave me the consciousness-shifting kick I'd been looking for. It yanked me straight into the present moment; for a few seconds, my thoughts were peaceful, my head felt light and a deep sense of joy rippled through my body. The effect was transformative and sustained. Hours later, I could feel it, and even now, as I write this, I can still feel that same refreshing sensation coursing through my body. And so, the next day, I was bitterly disappointed when I tried the organic kefir I'd bought from the supermarket to have at the clinic for lunch. It was barely sour at all, almost cloying – and incredibly dull. The experience reminded me just how vital our expectations of food are. If you're expecting a sweet milky drink and instead get something thick and sour, it's understandable to be annoyed. If you're expecting the refreshing sourness of kefir and end up with some sweet supermarket drink, disappointment is inevitable. In the hope of avoiding a repeat of this situation, I now own a special yoghurt and kefir maker. It retains heat like a vacuum flask, allowing me to achieve the level of fermentation I want by controlling the temperature.

For anyone who prefers to avoid milk products, water kefir – related to kombucha – is an easy way of producing probiotics in large quantities. You add kefir grains, sugar, lemon slices, dried figs and water to a fermenting jar and wait. Every day for four days, you pour off a small amount of the liquid, seal it in a jar in the fridge and let it cool before tasting it to check the fermentation process in real time. The more advanced fermentation becomes, the more the sweetness decreases and the more pronounced the refreshing, sour taste becomes. Time and again, making water kefir has proved to be a mindful experience for me and what I've learned is this: sugar is likeable enough, it has plenty of superficial charm, but in the long run it tempts you towards inertia, because it's simply nice and nothing more and offers no suggestions or stimuli of its own. In contrast, acids are a little unusual, seeming tight and aloof at first, but eventually they become your best friends, proving helpful in all sorts of situations.

But if you really can't see yourself warming to fermented foods, there are other, much simpler exercises to get you on your way. At the start of the week, slice up some lemons or limes and store them in an airtight container in the fridge. Have a taste now and again to remind yourself of their sour flavour. Ultimately, it's never too late to make friends with acidic foods.

Bitterness: the language of plants

Our next step is to use mindful eating to develop a taste for bitter foods. It's a unique challenge because bitter flavours can indicate the presence of both healthy antioxidants and toxins. Humans have been facing this challenge head-on for millennia, with chocolate, coffee and beer – all of them rich in bitter compounds – gaining tremendous popularity. We have successfully overcome one of the plant world's key protective measures, which has evolved hundreds of thousands of bitter compounds to deter hungry animals. Many of these substances were toxic at one time, but herbivorous animals have developed enzymes in their livers and cultivated bacteria in their guts that render these toxins harmless. Human beings have inherited these detoxification methods. Yet our methods are far from perfect, which is why we have retained a delicate sense of taste for bitterness, enabling us to assess the levels of toxins in foods before they are digested, spit them out if necessary and avoid them in the future.

If you look at the animal kingdom, the connection between bitterness and protection against poisoning reveals itself. Insectivorous frogs have the keenest and most refined sense when it comes to bitter flavours, because any insect they eat could well contain large quantities of toxins. Since toxicity has nothing to do with the shape or size of prey and everything to do with what it eats and the contents of its gut, frogs must carefully test the bitterness of any insect they happen to wrap their tongues around. At the other end of the spectrum, there are animals with no sense of bitterness, such as penguins and whales, which do not eat plants and tend to swallow their prey rather than chew it, leaving them no time to assess the taste on their tongues carefully. They can indulge in gobbling up prey without a care in the world because the crustaceans, squid, cuttlefish and schools of fish they feed on do not contain such toxins.

The evolution of higher animals and humankind reveals a curious change in these animals' sense of bitterness, despite this having proven a successful strategy for millions of years. The larger an animal's brain, the less likely it is to fear bitterness. This speaks to the fact that higher animals with greater intelligence, experience and the ability to exchange information were able to determine whether toxins were present without a sense of bitterness and, in doing so, discovered the existence of non-toxic bitter plants. But the truly groundbreaking discovery, which I call the bitter paradox, was ultimately made by apes. They recognised that bitter plants could have healing properties. It is well documented that African chimpanzees deliberately eat bitterleaf to kill off bothersome intestinal parasites. According to the bitter paradox, therefore, certain bitter plants are not only tolerable, they actually have health benefits which go far beyond their nutritional content. In a way, chimpanzees ought to be lauded as the founders of herbal medicine.

One of the many bitter plant substances with a vital part to play in modern medicine today is salicin, which is found in willow trees and is the active ingredient in aspirin, one of the most indispensable drugs we have, due to its ability to ease pain, lower fever, reduce inflammation and thin the blood. Other examples include papaverine, from the opium poppy, which relaxes the blood vessels and muscles in the event of colic or spasms, or the antimalarial quinine, derived from the bark of the cinchona tree and used to add bitterness in small quantities to drinks such as Bitter Lemon and Tonic Water.

Newborn babies have yet to realise the medicinal potential of bitter substances and prefer the sweet flavours they recognise from their mothers' milk, which is why they typically reject bitter foods. We have to learn to appreciate bitter flavours throughout our lives. The greater a child's fear of bitterness is, the harder it is to wean them. Some midwives even recommend turning children who are keen to continue nursing off the breast by applying mustard or bitter almond flavouring. An aversion to bitter foods can delay the broadening of a child's food spectrum, contributing to poor nutrition and eating disorders. A common casualty of this aversion is citrus fruit, which happens to be both sour and bitter, as well as exceptionally good for us. The same applies to vegetables, particularly spinach and Brussels sprouts, which children tend to avoid despite their health benefits. One way to gently introduce children to the world of healthy bitter foods is to offer them lightly roasted pine nuts and other such nuts.

Of course, looking beyond foods that happen to be both bitter and good for us, there are bitter substances that are toxic. Our sense of taste knows what it's doing when it warns us off the bitter taste of nicotine. No substance is as quick to become addictive as bitter tobacco. Green beans are another example; their bitter taste comes from toxic cyanhydric acid. A strong, bitter flavour suggests your beans were not cooked long enough. Then there's cassava, which has a highly toxic defence system to deter herbivores. However, when properly washed and peeled, cassava is a valuable staple, enjoyed by half a million people in the tropics. In this case, the tuber's bitterness helps us to assess how well it has been prepared. In antiquity, bitter poisons were used to kill people. Socrates, the famous ancient philosopher, accepted a death sentence rather than renounce his ideals of justice, choosing to drink a beaker of poison hemlock. The bitter substances in this pretty, harmless-looking umbellifer – found across Europe – gradually cause the victim to stop breathing. While the details surrounding Socrates' death remain hazy to this day, we know that he died fully conscious and with a bitter taste in his mouth.

You could almost go so far as to say that bitterness is an existential flavour. It leads us on a journey for just the correct dose, walking the line between a good life and utter ruin, between poison and cure. Due to this ambivalence, there are numerous connections between a person's love of bitterness and their personality. Bitter substances are stimulating, so it's no surprise that they are particularly popular with people who are curious, outgoing and open to new things. By contrast, people with an excessive love of bitter flavours, those for whom beer or chocolate can never be bitter enough, tend to lead embittered lives, exhibiting hostile, narcissistic and aggressive personality traits.[24] At the other end of the spectrum, some people prefer to combat any hint of bitterness with sweetness. They have the advantage of a lot of understanding for people who are sensitive and have no desire to endure the stress of bitterness. In my native German, we have the phrase 'süßes Nichtstun', literally 'sweet idleness', which may well allude to the connection between a love of sugar and the desire for a stress-free life devoid of bitterness.

The benefits of bitter substances are manifold and, to a large extent, still unknown. There's an old German adage: 'Bitter im Mund, Magen gesund'. You might translate it as, 'Bitterness on the tongue makes for a healthy tum'. Indeed, bitter substances support bowel function and the release of digestive juices. In the gut and the liver, bitter substances activate systems that reduce the intake of toxic substances and set the liver's detoxification processes in motion. Furthermore, certain bitter substances can reduce inflammation and have antimicrobial and antioxidative effects. This appears to explain the health benefits of olive oil. People in Italy's Blue Zones consume around half a litre of olive oil per week and live longer than Northern Europeans and Americans, who consume less. According to the large-scale PREDIMED study, olive oil and walnuts are the only superfoods to have a positive effect on blood fat and help prevent heart attacks, despite being almost pure fat themselves.

Unfortunately, the quality of olive oils varies considerably. However, mindful eating and drinking can help us choose the right kinds of oils. A peppery, bitter aftertaste in the back of your throat, perhaps prompting a slight cough, suggests that an olive oil contains plenty of healthy bitter substances. Other exciting bitter substances include catechins in green tea, which, according to new research, are not antioxidants but pro-oxidants. Much like vaccines, pro-oxidants strengthen the body's defensive capabilities, essentially by challenging them. It calls to mind the adage, 'What doesn't kill you makes you stronger.' As ever, the correct dose is crucial, so it's important not to drink too much green tea and green tea extracts or concentrates are best avoided. High doses of catechins impair the function of the mitochondria, the powerhouse of our bodies' cells, so severely that they can lead to cell death, particularly in the liver.[25] Thus, bitterness appears to have two things to teach us: one, that the world is full of danger, and two, that it's worth engaging with it anyway – albeit with caution not least because many dangers conceal new opportunities.

Germany was once home to a woman who discovered and wrote about the dangers but potential curative effects of bitterness. In the twelfth century, Hildegard von Bingen introduced bitterness to Germany and the Western world through her mystical writings and herbal medicine. Some details of her medical writings no longer stand up from a contemporary perspective, such as her belief that peaches, strawberries and figs were useless to the body or difficult to digest. Nevertheless, her work is full of surprises. It is not so much the medical aspect that shines through in her work as her captivating spirit, such as her unwavering devotion to those who sought her help and put their trust in her, even in the most difficult of situations.

As a psychiatrist, I am impressed by her matter-of-factness and neutrality, treating emotional problems (such as a lack of sexual desire) and psychological disturbances (such as frenzies of rage, madness and alcoholism) with the same level of dedication with which she treats physical conditions. It made no difference to Hildegard whether her patient was a man, woman, child, Christian, or Jew. She even granted animals her full attention and care. To judge or condemn any creature that was suffering was alien to her. Reading one of her works, *Physica*, I was overcome by the sense that I was not reading a medieval text so much as hearing a voice from the future.

In the Middle Ages, the theory of the four humours was at the foundation of all medical study. It harks back to the ancient Greek physician Hippocrates, who claimed that disease is caused by an imbalance of blood, phlegm, yellow bile and black bile. According to this theory, melancholics suffered from an excess of cold, black bile, cholerics had too much hot, yellow bile, phlegmatics were excessively 'moist' and bunged up with white phlegm and sanguine types were too 'dry', because their blood was boiling. Hildegard also subscribed to this theory and worked mainly as a dietary consultant. According to her, cholerics should avoid 'hot' spices, phlegmatics must be prescribed a diet of 'dry' dishes, melancholics ought to opt for warm, aromatic foods and sanguines are best off eating cold, moist fish. However, Hildegard was also brave and inspired enough to add a fifth, green element to this quartet of fluids, one that enabled her to lay the theoretical foundation for herbal medicine. She named it viriditas, after the Latin 'viridis' meaning 'green'. The term also alluded to the virility inherent in green bitterness, or virginity, emphasising the powers of renewal and rejuvenation inherent to herbal medicine. Hildegard also used viriditas in the sense of the Latin 'vis', emphasising vitality and potency and highlighting the unity and interdependence of humanity and nature.

From a contemporary perspective, in a society where Green politicians strive to reestablish the balance between humans and nature using renewable energy, Hildegard's concept of a greening power uniting plants, humanity and the cosmos seems almost prophetic. Hildegard also knew that the bitterness in plants could make food and drink last longer. Her concept of viriditas was both an advertisement for sustainability and a means of preventing food waste. The original, unhopped beer that people drank for thousands of years would spoil quickly, as the bacteria and wild yeasts in it multiplied. Not long before Hildegard's birth, German brewers began adding hops to beer to give it a longer shelf life. Hops are the female flowers of the hop vine and look like little pale green cones. Their oils inhibit microbial growth and give drinks a unique flavour with notes of geranium, pine and citrus, along with a hearty bitterness. Hildegard was so enthusiastic about this longer-lasting, hoppy beer that she lauded it as a veritable elixir. She was also smart enough to know that beer didn't suit everyone and made a point of warning her melancholic patients against using beer to lift their spirits. The bitterest beer on the market is India Pale Ale (IPA), which originated in the UK. It was initially brewed with large amounts of hops to preserve it during the long journey from India to England. I tried a particularly bitter variety called Avery India Pale Ale and the sharp, piney bitterness was so strong that my mouth dried up from shock.

Hildegard's practice of using bitter herbs to stimulate digestion and the production of digestive juices was further developed a few hundred years later in Rheinberg, to the north of the abbey where she lived, by the Underberg family, who continue to produce a popular brand of digestive bitters to this day. The drink invites you to experience the full, green vitality of nature, largely foregoing the mellowing taste of salt and the magic of umami. Unlike other bitter liquors, such as Fernet Branca and Unicum, it does not contain any refined sugars. Only five people worldwide are privy to the recipe, which remains a closely guarded secret. Take a mindful sip, however and it becomes clear that the basis of the drink is some grain-based spirit, flavoured with a variety of herbs. The herbs themselves are said to come from forty-three different countries. I would hazard a guess that they include fennel and aniseed, a little ginger and liquorice and perhaps a touch of nettle, which Hildegard recommended for cleansing the stomach. The absence of refined sugars, which curtails bitter flavours, allows that bright greenness to hit with full effect, radiating from your mouth across your face and eventually reaching the top of your skull. In a flash, it was clear to me why Hildegard was so convinced that bitter flavours (such as radish, for instance) cleansed the brain.

The Ayurveda confirms that Vata types like myself enjoy a touch of stimulating bitterness, but warns against overdoing it. Hildegard herself takes the same line, arguing that the bitterness of any medicine ought to be adjusted to the sensitivities of the person being treated. Despite this sensible advice, I can't help but continue making a daily trip to the mildly bitter world of tea. I've been drinking it for decades, out of the same green cup. I feel that the bitter flavours have built up inside it over the years and have become more refined. I almost always start my day with the earthy, fruity bitterness of an English Breakfast Tea. Its warm, malty flavours muffle its bitter ingredients and offer a touch of protection against the bitterness of life. On occasion, I'll choose a Japanese green tea, such as a Sencha Yamato. The leaves are harvested young and I let them brew for a mere twenty seconds before drinking. This tea has a lightness and freshness and its flavour, like cut grass, can awaken childhood memories and feelings of security, helping me feel in touch with myself and strengthening my intuition. Later in the morning, I enjoy the refined bitter flavours of Earl Grey, scented with citrussy bergamot. I save the Eastern spiritual bitterness of Darjeeling – the Champagne of teas – for the afternoon. I take pleasure in observing how its light, fruity flavours intermingle with its darker, musky ones. Finally, when bedtime beckons, I reach for a cup of verbena tea; I love its gentle bitterness, evoking hints of lemon, mint and mandarin. The German name for verbena, *Eisenkraut* (literally 'iron herb'), harks back to the age of chivalry, when verbena was used to treat wounds made by iron weapons. It is what makes it so well-suited to cleaning away the scars and the sickness of the day.

The less fermented a tea is, the more umami flavours it will contain, thereby softening its bitterness. White tea is the least fermented and therefore the least bitter, followed by green tea, blue Oolong and black tea, which, depending on the variety, exudes an earthy bitterness. You can also adjust bitterness with brewing time: the shorter the brew, the less bitter the tea. All the tea varieties I have listed are comparable in terms of their anti-inflammatory and antioxidative effects. Green tea also contains pro-oxidants, while black tea contains more caffeine. Unlike these teas, which all come from the tea plant, herbal teas are much more diverse. Chamomile tea, for instance, has hardly any bitterness at all when brewed for a short time. It's good for soothing irritation in the mouth and airways. Wormwood tea is the most bitter tea I have come across, but it can work wonders for loss of appetite, digestive issues and bad breath.

To better get to know the greening power local to me, I took my old schoolmate, Marc Germann, on a trip to the Reichenbach Falls in the Bernese Oberland. The location itself is not exactly known for being home to healing plants and herbs. Still, thanks to Arthur Conan Doyle's Sherlock Holmes story, *The Final Problem*, it has become a popular tourist destination. Doyle describes the bitter struggle between Holmes and his archenemy, Professor Moriarty, which ends with the two of them falling into the gorge below. It is, therefore, the location of the archetypal battle between powers that heal and powers that harm, which, in my view, makes it an ideal place to learn to distinguish good bitter tastes from potentially harmful ones. Marc studied geography and also trained to be a farmer. He led me through wild mountain meadows, where we gazed in wonder at the vast diversity of different plants and herbs: sage, thyme, peppermint, ribwort plantain, elderflowers in bloom, fragrant mosses and much more besides. I was intent on diving in and giving each plant a taste without much ado. Marc didn't think this was advisable, but he didn't try to stop me, trusting that I would soon come to recognise which plants would do me good and which would not. Taste plays a vital role in categorising plants – look no further than their names: *bitter*cress, *sour*grass, *sweet* cicely. I wasn't the first to be using my tongue to explore the world of plants, rather than just my nose and eyes. I bit into juicy, bitter valerian roots, the bitter leaves of St John's wort, I enjoyed the sour taste of young clover and the delicate flavour notes of six-sided stonecrop. I noticed that almost all the plants were bitter, but in their own unique ways. The way I experienced it, Hildegard's greening power was bitter.

Nevertheless, my experiment came to an abrupt end when I found myself chewing on a small piece of an unremarkable, egg-shaped leaf. Suddenly, waves of bitterness overcame me. I felt dizzy and sick and my whole body tensed up. I spat out the leaf straight away, but my mouth seemed to have become a single, pulsing glob of bitterness. It was as if I had eaten a magic mushroom; I lost myself for a moment, not to a sense of relaxation, but to a sense of fear – and stomach cramps. Using a plant identification app, Marc eventually worked out that I had taken a bite of wild lettuce. Its German name, *Giftlattich*, or 'poison lettuce', did little to reassure me. Fortunately, wild lettuce is only harmful to human beings in large quantities. I had finally experienced the darker side of bitterness for myself. Even so, the experience – one our nomadic ancestors would have had fairly often – was very interesting. I experienced the vast breadth of bitterness; not just the taste, but how long it lasted and the sensations it provoked, the indications that poison was present.

Craving heat

Our love of hot and spicy foods is psychologically related to our penchant for bitter flavours. Again, it's curious, risk-taking and occasionally non-conformist individuals who tend to feel the desire for spice most keenly. Biologically speaking, our ability to perceive spice is in a world of its own. We do not use our sense of taste to detect hot spice; instead, it is our senses of pain and temperature that do the heavy lifting, via our skin, tongues and mouths. These sensations travel to the brain via the trigeminal nerve, named for its three branches. The uppermost branch leads to the eyes, the middle branch leads to the upper jaw and the bottom leads to the lower jaw. Unlike our sense of taste, which passively experiences flavours and transmits them, stimulation of the trigeminal nerve causes pain. When this reaction occurs, the tongue serves as the alarm control panel, responding like a concerned *maître d'* at a restaurant, running from one table to the next to check if everything is OK. Encountering a fiery and furious customer, or one with a sharp tongue, he raises the alarm. He knows these kinds of patrons can do lasting damage to the whole restaurant, which, for this analogy, is the oral mucous membrane and the digestive system. Emergency measures are deployed, including a massive increase in mental focus, sweat and plenty of saliva to clean the mouth; vomiting and diarrhoea can also follow in an attempt to cleanse the whole digestive tract. The trigeminal nerve is also responsible for the eyes, which start to water. Spicy foods can even cause unpleasant sensations in the anus and the vagina, as these body parts also have heat receptors.

As soon as the mouth has been cleared of its troublesome customers, a second, curious reaction occurs, one which is particularly significant in the world of medicine: areas of the tongue which have come into contact with the spicy food turn numb. It is suspected that this allows us to use the higher centres of the brain to consciously determine whether the tongue has overreacted, enabling us to eat more of the spicy dish with a numb tongue if necessary. This allows us to eat lots of plants that animals do not like. The disadvantage is that a numb tongue can cause human beings to ingest poison in large quantities. In the age of ubiquitous supermarkets, however, it's a manageable risk. The painfully spicy foods on offer pose no danger to us.

What's particularly interesting is the pain we experience when eating chilli peppers, which, depending on the degree of spiciness, equates to a false alarm. How did an error of this kind find its way into our personal alert system? Plants are incredibly clever. Rooted to the spot, they communicate via chemical substances which can attract, repel, or poison animals. The chemistry of plants is so ingenious that it produces substances capable of outwitting the nervous systems of animals and human beings. One of its most remarkable success stories is the chemical capsaicin, which gives chilli peppers, wasabi and ginger their spicy heat. Capsaicin triggers the mouth's alert system without being poisonous. At some point in the past, certain danger-loving human beings discovered that chilli peppers and wasabi activated the body's pain system, but that it was possible to become accustomed to the burning sensation that ensued, only to be rewarded with a healthy dose of endorphins. Endorphins are the body's own painkillers. The brain assumes severe damage to the mouth and mobilises what the body needs to survive. Yet endorphins don't just relieve pain, they also provoke a warm feeling of trust and connectedness. There's a lot to be said for spicy heat.

In Chinese, the numbing effect of some spices is known as 'mala'. In Sichuan province, it is used to create a unique taste experience. Sichuan pepper numbs the mouth, allowing other spicy flavours in a dish to shine with greater nuance and distinction, fostering a mindful, pleasurable eating experience. Incidentally, Sichuan pepper is not related to black pepper; it is derived from the spicy, aromatic seed pods of an Asian citrus fruit. In one of my own experiments with Sichuan pepper, I discovered that the pain I felt was accompanied by a narcotic warmth which spread throughout my whole body. In this respect, I can understand why American authorities classified Sichuan pepper as a drug from 1968 to 2005, outlawing it for years. Yet most of the available Sichuan peppers are disappointingly harmless. Only very fresh, high-quality pepper has the desired numbing and warming effects.

The numbing effects of pepper have also been used in medicine. Capsaicin in chilli peppers has been used for pain relief, for instance, in pain relief patches and creams to treat shingles and muscle aches. Menthol, found in mint and camphor, is capsaicin's baby brother. It offers similar numbing effects, but without causing acute pain. It also creates a cooling sensation without being cold, just as chilli peppers and wasabi prompt a feeling of sweat-inducing heat despite not being hot. Plant chemistry fools our bodies' sense of temperature and we're happy for it to do so.

As well as these psychological and culinary effects, our love of spicy heat also has more tangible consequences, such as ensuring our survival. Hot spices are particularly popular in warmer countries, where people are more exposed to harmful bacteria, because they can use their herbal arsenal to kill disease-causing bacteria. It's no accident that curry was invented in India and not Finland. Spices are made from the toughest parts of fruits and vegetables, which is why they contain such high levels of antimicrobial compounds. It wasn't gold that Columbus was searching for on his voyages so much as cinnamon, cloves and pepper. In 1492, these spices were far more valuable than any precious metal.

Mindfully and gradually developing our sense of spicy heat is a way to discover new culinary possibilities and to exercise restraint over our desire for that spicy kick. Hot spices also curb appetite and boost metabolism, which can help with weight loss.

Eating and eroticism: tingling, moistening, contracting

Our mouths are where we make physical contact with

our food. It's why they have touch receptors, as well as all the other receptors we have discussed. This sense of touch tells us how hard, soft, dry, or fluid the food we have chewed is and conveys to us the tingling sensation in a glass of Champagne. It is also an important part of eroticism, which explains why many people find cooking and eating erotic. In antiquity, a love of licking and tasting, salt, spice and unusual flavours was seen as proof that someone was good in bed. Culinary and erotic desire also often coincide in the Bible. There are erotic undertones to Eve's seducing Adam to taste the apple in the Garden of Eden, and these same undertones are echoed in the Song of Songs: 'Your lips drip nectar, my bride; honey and milk are under your tongue; the fragrance of your garments is like the fragrance of Lebanon.' The Indian sages also recognised the deep connection between food and sex, grounded in touch and mindful eating. An Indian poem written in the Middle Ages reads: 'Your breath is like honey, spiced with cloves; your mouth is delicious like a ripe mango. The deep hollow of your navel harbours delicacies. Only the tongue knows the pleasures of resting within them, though it can never tell.'

The tongue could tell us one thing, though and that is that passion has a lot to do with the right amount of fluid. A dry mouth is not particularly sexy, nor is an excess of drool – perhaps because both conditions could point to a problem with the digestive tract, a complex system tasked with supplying the world within our bodies with the right amount of juice. Curiously, when it comes to the erotic, medical terminology is forever throwing up terms that couldn't be less sexy if they tried: 'sialagogic', for instance, refers to something which promotes the flow of saliva. Sweet treats of all kinds encourage saliva production and good bread should turn moist in the mouth. The opposite of this term is the word 'astringent', which refers to something which causes the mouth to contract and dry out. Milk, coffee, black tea, green tea, red wine and fruit all dry out the mouth because they contain tannins. Tannins bind to proteins in our saliva, inhibiting its flow.

Sudden moisture is an unmistakable sign of arousal. The Chilean writer Isabel Allende writes of the following experience in her book, *Aphrodite*: 'No one who has lived to adulthood and has held a fresh tomato in the palm of his hand and bitten into it, feeling its flesh in his mouth as juice streams down his chin, can escape the temptation to compare it with other oral pleasures.'[26]

In her autobiography, the American author Judith Moore describes eating a cake, its sweetness making her salivate and arousing mystical feelings: 'The first bite rises toward the opening mouth. The sentinel nose, having anticipated pie's arrival, a tide of saliva crests in the mouth, pools in the tongue's centre and washes over the several thousand taste buds. The teeth bite through a flaky, slightly salty crust, then into tart cherries, rhubarb and apple. The fruits' sweet, buttery juices, in a total-immersion baptism of the mouth, flood the tongue, teeth and cheeks. There is no more outside. Everything is in.'[27]

Our bodies have specialised sensors for detecting mechanical stimuli, known as end-organ mechano-receptors. These respond to moisture and temperature and can be found in the mucous membranes of the lips and tongue, but also on the penis and clitoris. They are the most direct proof that food and the erotic are connected. A friend of mine claims she and her husband have always suspected that their genitals have a sense of taste. They use pomegranate oil as a lubricant. When it comes to long-lasting passion, the balance between moisture and dryness is crucial. The Bible typically recommends that two foods be eaten together to foster love. In the Old Testament, it is mouthwatering honey and drying milk; in the New Testament, it is moist bread and dry wine. In France, the baguette, a Parisian favourite, combines both elements. The outside should be dry and crisp and the inside should be moist and spongy. Red wine is a recommended accompaniment to coq au vin and ossobuco because both are oily dishes bathed in their own juices and the astringent, drying effect of red wine prevents the palate from being overwhelmed. In contrast, fish is commonly served alongside a glass of white wine because the latter draws no moisture from the fish, letting it swim along happily. In Italy, risotto combines soft, creamy elements with al dente rice, which offers a slight resistance to the dish's liquid elements.

The well-practised tongue mentioned above could also have plenty to tell us about the specific qualities of certain juices, like the tingling sensation, that tickly, stimulating feeling that is apt to transform a desire for individual nutrients into an all-round sensory delight.

At orgies in Ancient Rome, whole baths would be filled with sparkling wine to make the passions of the men and women romping about inside them extra pleasurable. In the present day, mineral water and carbonated fizzy drinks allow us to integrate that tingling, tickly feeling into our otherwise rather buttoned-up daily working lives, restricting it to our mouths.

The well-practised tongue might also reveal secrets about higher forms of pleasure, which are always bound up with action. The Arabic erotic manual, *The Perfumed Garden of Sensual Delight*, says: 'Woman is like a fruit, which will not yield its sweetness until you rub it between your hands. Look at the basil plant; if you do not rub it warm with your fingers it will not emit any scent.'[28] This erotic guide is also an instruction manual for mindful eating: the tongue must invest in pleasure. The Greek philosopher Plato saw things the same way. For Plato, higher forms of eroticism and spirituality were characterised by the fact that they did not simply passively receive impressions of beauty but actively produced it. The same applies to higher forms of mindful eating, in which beauty can be experienced through careful touching, moistening and chewing. Sensual eating requires the tongue to put in the effort, but it also requires time. It's hardly surprising that it was the puritanical Americans who invented the almost untranslatable terms 'snack' and 'quickie'. It's equally unsurprising that Americans live on average seven years fewer than the inhabitants of the Blue Zones, who have fully committed themselves to mindful, pleasure-filled eating and slow eroticism.

The well-practised tongue would undoubtedly tell us that, from time to time, it is permissible and even necessary to make noise. Some Middle Eastern texts state that a kiss should make a sound, producing a light, long-lasting sound between the tongue and the moist edge of the palate. The sucking movement of the tongue in the mouth causes an audible displacement of saliva. You might interpret this as a guide to mindful lip-smacking and slurping on an oil-slicked plate of pasta or a seafood soup, full of the scents and flavours of the sea. Losing yourself in a lip-smacking meal is proof of a relaxed relationship with pleasure and physicality.

We could also ask the well-practised tongue about aphrodisiacs, i.e. means of increasing erotic passion. For some time, erotic foods have been viewed as medicines possessing specific ingredients for stimulating the libido. Yet modern science disagrees. Even bull testicles and sage tea – which the ancient Greeks are said to have given soldiers returning home to boost their potency and shore up the Greek population against extinction – are astonishingly ineffective chemically. The well-practised tongue might reveal to us, then, that the secret of aphrodisiacs lies in their sensory effects, stimulating our imaginations via our senses of sight, touch and smell. Writers of every era have compared the human body to foods to emphasise its eroticism: whipped cream for a fresh-looking complexion, ripe peaches for soft cheeks and red cherries for kissable lips. Madame du Barry, one of history's most notorious seductresses, dosed her 'victims' – including the French King Louis XV – with a blend of egg yolk and ginger to give them ravenous sexual appetites. In the Tantric tradition, sweet and universally popular bananas form the bridge between food and eroticism. Isabel Allende recommends that her lovers feed her crisp, cooling cucumbers to stir her appetite. In turn, Allende presents potential lovers with fresh oysters, not to arouse them but to test and train their erotic capabilities. Typically, fruits and seashells are popular symbols of the female genitalia because they share the same inviting moistness and tart astringency. Quinces are the fruit of Aphrodite, the Greek goddess of sensual desire. In Italy, figs represent the vulva, while the symbolic fruits of choice in China are plums and peaches. Erotic desire stirs, to a significant degree, in the mouth and mindful eating allows us to foster and guide that desire.

There is a direct link between oral eroticism and herbal medicine. Hildegard von Bingen divided the curative effects of foods into four categories: cold, warm, moist and dry. These categories are generally interpreted in a spiritual sense, corresponding to the four elements of air, fire, water and earth. Yet Hildegard repeatedly indicated that the taste of these remedies was also crucial to her, contradicting the idea that a spiritual interpretation is the only valid one. She must have been influenced in her work as a healer by the day-to-day experiences of having bread turn moist in her mouth, red wine drying her tongue, pepper bringing her out in a sweat and mint offering cooling refreshment. It was proof that foods have a physiological impact which does not stem from temperature or water content. These experiences with taste could explain why certain principles of Hildegard's medicinal thinking have endured to this day. Among them are the practice of using cooling menthol and camphor to cool a hot, inflamed joint, or using spicy ginger and nettle to warm up a leg suffering from poor circulation. Astringent tannins from sage, bay and other medicinal plants help to reduce excess saliva production and treat excessive blood flow in cases of gingivitis, eczema, or even open wounds. Mucous-promoting salt and soothing chamomile are a proven treatment for rehydrating mucous membranes.

Mystical eating

On sabbatical in New York in the spring of 2016, I had a curious experience. One morning, as every morning, I was queuing at a café on the Upper East Side, where my family and I lived. A group of women was ahead of me in the queue; a modelling agency was nearby and these women may have been models from that agency. I watched as they all bought a single chocolate bar each. They unwrapped the bars and bit off a piece, chewing it mindfully, slowly and with pleasure, breathing deeply as they did so. And then they spat out the chocolate. They threw the rest of the bar in the bin, keeping the wrapper so that they could breathe in the chocolatey smell with something approaching a wild fervour. I was astonished. A man standing nearby piped up: 'That's mystical eating.' He explained that mystical eating was a way to suppress hunger without having to avoid sweets altogether. Only much later did I manage to understand these women and their 'mystical eating'; it wasn't just a strange display of behaviour, it could have been an indicator of a severe eating disorder.

As a psychiatrist, I can't recommend this kind of behaviour, but it does remind me that scent and our sense of smell play an essential role in mindful eating and I've neglected this thus far. I hope to demonstrate that the complexity of olfactory perception can evoke mystical feelings and states of being – perhaps these were what those women sought, just in an unhealthy way. So, here are the basics: we have two senses of smell. The first is our ability to sniff out the world around us. It allows us to evaluate foods, people and air quality. Is this person familiar or a stranger? Are they good or bad? Dogs and rodents are vastly superior to us in this respect, most likely because we walk upright, our noses are higher up and we experience the world around us primarily through our eyes. Still, that's no reason to conclude that we have poor noses overall. The models in New York didn't sniff at their chocolate wrappers like dogs following a scent; instead, they breathed the aroma in deeply. This is where our second sense of smell comes in, helping us to assess a scent using our mouths. This is known as retronasal olfaction (from the

Latin 'retro' for 'behind'). The flavours do not stream in through the nose; instead, they rise from the back of the mouth past the back of the nose. We are world champions when it comes to exploring the scent of our own mouths and guts, because, compared to other animals, our noses are much more open than our oral cavities.

Here's a simple way to experience retronasal olfaction. Close your eyes, pinch your nose and select a gummy bear from a packet and chew it without looking. Your tongue will immediately tell you that you have something sweet in your mouth, but you won't be able to tell what flavour the gummy bear is. Only once you give your nostrils free rein will the fruity flavour reveal itself. And the scent you experience will be more precise and more intense than if you were to sniff the gummy bear. This is because retronasal olfaction is more sensitive than our immune systems, requiring fewer molecules to create a scent than to activate our immune systems. A mindful person's retronasal olfactory faculties can pick up the tiniest hints of cyanide in bitter almonds, even though their immune system would not react to it. Our brains assess the air we inhale according to strict rules about possible dangers and the potential benefits of environmental stimuli. These include social smells and environmental smells such as smoke, gas and decay. Exhaled air enters through the back of the nose, receiving sophisticated processing in the highest regions of the cerebral cortex. This is why smells can evoke complex feelings and memories. In the Upanishads, a series of

Hindu mystical texts, all spiritual teachings, myths, stories, mystical insights and their interpretations are understood as an exhalation of the self. Indeed, when we exhale, our food becomes part of us, our stories and our culture. The experience of retronasal olfaction is at the heart of Marcel Proust's epoch-defining novel *À la recherche du temps perdu [In Search of Lost Time]*. The taste of a madeleine dunked in tea reminds the narrator of his childhood, serving as the catalyst for the subsequent tale, which spans over four thousand pages. Today, the Proust effect is the name given to the phenomenon whereby specific surroundings can stir up intense memories, a tree, perhaps, a place, a person, or a food that transports us back to the past. Scent often plays an integral part in this because it has the most immediate access to unconscious traces of memory. In the Hindu scriptures, retronasal olfaction possesses a mystical quality, as different times and places blend. *Is that scent coming from my body or from outside of it? Am I sensing it in my mouth or in my nose? Am I experiencing something in my immediate surroundings or from my past?* This mysterious expansion of consciousness is temporary and can suddenly take on a deeper meaning. All these are also characteristics of the mystical state.

Thanks to our skills of retronasal olfaction, no animal, not even a bloodhound, can beat us when it comes to distinguishing between different scents. Early man was a nomadic omnivore, for whom distinguishing edible from poisonous foods was essential across various locations and times. Eventually, human beings began to process, grill and cook foods, as well as making them last longer through fermentation. Our retronasal sense of smell helped us develop these methods, retain them in memory and test their usefulness. Thus, mindful eating is much more than just a way of controlling our weight – it's a central component of human culture and evolution.

The complex sensations that arise from exchanges of flavours, scents, visual and emotional information in the insular cortex, which reach consciousness as unified experiences, are known as olfactory images. The interplay between taste experiences is comparable to painting with opaque gouache. No new 'colours' of taste arise, but one taste will lessen or heighten another; sweet will soften bitter, while spicy tastes will strengthen bitter ones. By contrast, the interplay between scents is like painting with watercolours, with the thousands of different scents that our brains pick up giving rise to brand new 'colours'. Our scent receptors are stimulated not so much by the type of substance as by its vibrations. Each substance typically activates several receptors at once, much like a pianist playing a chord – except on an enormous keyboard. For example, a banana contains 300 flavour substances, a tomato contains 400 and coffee has no fewer than 600. There is a mystical quality to olfactory images and flavour music: mindfulness and mental openness expand consciousness to include new colours and sounds. The COVID-19 pandemic demonstrated just how vital these worlds are. Viral infections can cause a loss of smell. The opaque colours remain, but the watercolours are lost, which for many people results in a severe reduction in quality of life.

Another of the mystical qualities associated with smell stems from the fact that we have no precise language to describe it. Olfactory states, much like mystical states, are to some extent unspeakable and in-commnicable. In English, there are few words beyond 'smelly' for describing a scent more accurately. 'Nice smelling' and 'bad smelling' are more judgmental than they are descriptive. All the other words for fragrances are borrowed, typically from the origin of the scent (for instance 'rose-scented'), the chemical process that produces the scent (e.g. 'rotten', 'spoiled', or 'mouldy') or the mental response the scent invokes (such as 'nauseating' or 'refreshing'). We also use terms relating to our sense of taste for smells (such as 'sweet', 'sour' and 'bitter') or general notions of sensory qualities (such as 'balsamic', 'homely', or 'heavenly'). We could effortlessly pick out our own grandmother in a room full of grandmothers, but that doesn't mean that we'd be able to explain how we managed it. Our understanding of a person's facial expressions is largely unconscious, and the same applies to scents. It's easy enough to say that we recognise one smell or another and we might be able to link it to Italian cooking, or Indian cuisine, but we get stuck when we're expected to describe it in more concrete terms. That sense of something incomprehensible and inexpressible, connecting us for a fleeting moment to a larger context, is also found in mysticism.

Despite the absence of language, it is worth trying

to describe and understand scents to increase the mindfulness with which we interact with the world and activate the whole brain. Tip the tea leaves into a preheated cup, then breathe in their scent. *Is that wild honey, vanilla, lemon peel, plum jam? A bitter hint of nettle?* Let's think beyond foods here and be open to all kinds of scents. Does it smell like your grandfather's attic? Like the field where you played football as a kid? Like your mum's leather jacket? Like the jungle you once tramped your way through? Connections like these are what make enjoying food a uniquely personal experience.

Experimental types might like to try the Air Up bottle to explore the magic of retronasal scent perception. When you take a sip from the Air Up bottle, gas-based aromatic substances enter your mouth and travel up through the back of your nose. The effect is striking: you're drinking plain water, but the gas-based aromatic substances (which smell like lemon, orange, watermelon, peach, coconut, iced coffee, cola, or Red Bull) make it feel like you are experiencing them in your mouth and your throat rather than in your nose.

With all this at the back of your mind, it's much easier to understand the curious behaviour exhibited by those women in New York. By chewing a tiny piece of their favourite chocolate, they activated their retronasal scent perception, refreshing and strengthening the memory of the chocolate in their minds. Afterwards, all they needed to do was give the wrapper a sniff from time to time to awaken the memory and enjoy the mystical feelings the chocolate imparted, without worrying about the calories. This may be indicative of an eating disorder, but it helps us to understand Sister André's harmless weakness for baked Alaska. This seemingly improbable dessert, which combines hot and cold, works because the air bubbles in the meringue insulate the ice cream from the heat. Sister André probably enjoyed the mystical retronasal effect created by the gas-based scents in the bubbles, which is why she could enjoy such a small portion of her favourite dish. It calls to mind the bread that Jesus broke into small pieces; thanks to the diverse aromas contained within its airy pores, its retronasal effects would have pointed to a higher world.

Scent perception plays a vital role in many spiritual traditions beyond Christianity. Scents connect us not only to food, but also to ourselves, our own smells, our microbiome, as well as other people, nature, flowers, trees, meadows and animals. This connection is not limited to the nose; our whole bodies are involved, because every one of our cells possesses scent receptors, particularly those in the gut and brain. Scent is an essential part of our being-in-the-world. These days, we live in a visually oriented culture; our sense of sight is the best match for our rational, technical view of the world. Screens increasingly dominate our consciousness and we even conceive of time in images, as short or long. With sight, however, there is a clear boundary between inside and outside, between the self and the world. By contrast, scent perception is an intense, direct, emotional and intuitive complement and alternative to modern notions of space and time. Mindful eating and smelling present a wonderful opportunity for getting back into your body when you're stuck in your head. The Buddhist monk Thích Nhất Hạnh emphasised food's capacity to help us connect: 'In my tradition, we concentrate on food and look at it as we would the cosmos ... When you chew a piece of bread mindfully, without thinking, you understand what the bread contains within it. And that is why, when you mindfully chew a piece of bread, you are truly connected to the fullness of life.'[29]

I was introduced to mindful eating by my grandfather. He worked as a taster for a Swiss chocolate factory, helping to develop new products and improve on the existing ones by testing chocolate, truffles and biscuits and writing reports on them. I was always impressed when he would proudly show me the latest truffles his company had produced. He would draw my attention to the colours and sheen of the packaging, which subtly prepared the consumer for the contents within. He told me to listen carefully as he opened the packet because, to his mind, the sound it made was proof of the product's freshness. Once the packet was open, he would gaze, enthralled, at the positioning of the chocolates inside the box. He likened them to precious stones mounted on rings. Together we would breathe in the scent of the truffles and observe their delicate shells. And then, slowly, he would take one out and hold it to the light like a diamond, so that I could see the subtle decoration on its surface, gaze in awe at its elegant lines or its perfect round shape. Finally, he would let me bite off a tiny piece of the truffle and let it sit on my tongue. Chewing was strictly forbidden to give my mouth time to appreciate the full flavour of the truffle, feeling it, tasting it and smelling it. Next, he would have me chew the chocolate twice, so that the filling could make complete contact with the rest of my mouth. Together, we experienced how the flavour intensified and enjoyed the adventure of the chocolate's changing texture. After that, my grandfather would give the signal and it was time to swallow and we would observe how the sweet mass slipped from our mouths and down into our stomachs. And then, it was time to assess how long the aftertaste lasted. Was it just a brief, fleeting kick, a sugary prank, a cheap trick? Or did the truffle have the potential to create a more profound sense of satiety and contentment? Did it generate a joyfulness greater than itself? A sense of pleasure at the sweetness of life, at communion and fusion?

Using mindful eating to take back control of nutrition

The food industry – along with restaurants, television and smartphones – distracts us from a more conscious eating practice, which can lead to poor dietary choices and overeating. Mindful eating can help us regain control over our nutrition amid a whirlpool of developments which are detrimental to our health. Sister André, Kane Takana and Grandma Anna demonstrate the enormous potential of this mindfulness practice, as do the many people in the Blue Zones who eat for pleasure and live to grand old ages.

Isabel Allende writes about the aforementioned French Paradox: 'the French eat sitting down, with calm, enjoying each mouthful. Watching a bourgeois couple in a provincial bistro is a most instructive lesson: they dine ritually, in silence, concentrating on their food and drink, unaware of the rest of the universe. Their menu is varied, the portions small and they do not eat at all hours of the day and night. One keyword defines the French paradox: moderation.' This moderation holds that eating ought to be a form of self-observation. To do this, we have to sit upright at a table, switching off all screens and the radio. From time to time, it is good practice to eat alone and in silence.

Similarly, we should not let hunger tempt us into gobbling down food without thinking. Thích Nhất Hạnh often spoke of hunger as a crying baby, which was trying to get our attention: 'When a baby cries, its mother takes it in her arms and immediately tries to comfort it. By choosing to take a few breaths, we can recognise and accept our desire, putting a stop to the autopilot within that would reach straight for a bag of crisps.' It is only when we eat slowly that we give our bodies a chance to respond to what we are eating. It's no trivial thing. When we drink water, our thirst disappears in an instant. An energy drink may give us wings for a moment or two, but the physiological effects we purport to experience in both circumstances are impossible. It takes at least thirty minutes for water and sugar to reach the brain. What we experience is simply psychological: we are mentally anticipating the effects. Mindfulness involves recognising this sense of anticipation as an illusion and relying on what our bodies are saying and what we are immediately experiencing.

The food and drink we consume ought not to be too cold. The colder a food is, the less we can taste and smell it and the more challenging it becomes to eat mindfully. This is why restaurants hoping to shift large quantities of food serve icy drinks and why the food is generally colder than it would be at a gourmet restaurant, where there is no correlation between quantity and price. As a rule, we should try to keep track of what we eat. The more often we eat and the larger and more varied the portions, the harder it is for us to gauge how many calories we have consumed in a day. This particularly applies to people who are overweight, as they tend to eat larger portions more frequently and while distracted. By contrast, small and manageable portions place hunger and flavour perception at the heart of the eating experience.

The Oryoki eating ritual practised in Zen monasteries also highlights the importance of modest portions and can be traced back to the Buddha and the mendicants. This ritual is intended to maintain a monk's mindfulness around receiving, appreciating and consuming food. Tellingly, the ritual does not take place in a dining room but in a meditation hall. At the beginning of the ritual, all participants receive an Oryoki set comprising three stacking bowls, a wooden fork, a pair of chopsticks and a small spatula for scraping the bowls. The set is intended as a reminder that mendicants, or beggar monks, possess nothing more than their clothes and their bowls, which they use to beg for food. The participants sit in a meditative pose, waiting to present their empty bowls to the servers. This phase of the ceremony sees the master place precisely the right amount of food in the participants' bowls, ensuring there is no waste and no harm to their health. The participants then eat in silence to boost their awareness. After the bowls have been washed, some of the water used to clean them is drunk and the rest is collected and poured onto the garden. Nothing is to be wasted.

But you don't need laborious ceremonies to improve your sense of self-observation when you eat. It can be enhanced simply by focusing on the extensive sensory impressions that I have already described. *Am I helping my vagus nerve by pausing between bites and taking relaxed breaths? Am I consciously aware of the flavours in the dish I'm eating? Does my food contain sweet, salty, sour, bitter and umami flavours? How does the food feel? Is it crispy, crunchy, grainy, slimy, or moist? How does it sound when I chew? Is the food dehydrating or spicy?* These are the kinds of questions we can ask to regain control over the salt and sugar we eat, as well as all the other flavours and really use our sensory organs to gauge the portion size we need. A sip of water before or while eating can help sharpen our taste buds. Capsules of micronutrients and processed liquid meals are not suitable for mindful eating. They disrupt the experience of direct contact with food and nutrients because they pass through the mouth and oesophagus too quickly. We need every part of our digestive system and all its helpers to be able to assess foods, from our eyes, our hands and our noses, to our mouths, stomachs and guts, all the way down to our anuses.

MICROFASTING AND MACROFASTING

Slowing down and practising conscious awareness are at the heart of mindful eating. I intend to devote more time to these two topics in this chapter on fasting. Every meal is a challenge for the body, which mobilises various mechanical, biochemical, bacterial and hormonal systems to convert foods into usable nutrients. As we will see in the following chapter, this entails far more than just chemically breaking foods down into individual calories; it is a multi-level, creative process through which new nutrients and new compounds of nutrients emerge. A large portion of our brainpower is spent anticipating future events because the human organism functions better when it can prepare. This also applies to digestion. The great advantage of fixed mealtimes over irregular eating habits, then, is that the body is better able to brace itself to take in food. This manifests as the release of small doses of digestive hormones that help monitor hunger and prevent fat deposits from forming. By contrast, spontaneous snacking results in an excessive insulin dose because the body is caught off guard. Much like unexpected psychological stress, this contributes towards creating a sense of ravenous appetite and disgruntlement. Digestion is also an energy-intensive process and our bodies must use breaks in eating to regenerate and detoxify. Breaks in eating offer protection against various diseases and conditions such as obesity, diabetes, autoimmune diseases, bowel cancer and cardiac and circulatory problems. Periods of abstinence also increase sensitivity in the mouth and gut, making food taste better and mindful, conscious eating easier.

Fasting has a long history. First and foremost, it refers to the regular daily breaks in eating, as seen in the English and French words 'breakfast' and 'déjeuner'. Both terms mean 'to break a fast', which indicates that both languages consider a night's sleep a fast. I call these breaks micro-fasts to distinguish them from macro-fasting over a more extended period. Sister André, Kane Tanaka and Grandma Anna were committed and disciplined micro-fasters.

All methods of fasting emphasise the importance of a fixed daily routine. Even the oldest lifeforms on Earth – such as polyps or sponges, which consist of little more than a gut – were able to recognise the cycle of day and night and adjust their digestion to specific mealtimes. The first 'sensory organs' to emerge in these primitive creatures were cells sensitive to light and taste on the surface of their gut. These cells are linked to our retinas and our sense of taste. Adjusting digestive preparedness to the time of day was the first indispensable step in excellent life optimisation. Fasting activates a kind of primaeval saving plan, making it ideal for regaining a sense of rhythm and energy during chaotic phases of life. In the Bible, King David fasted to weather political crises and survive the deaths of his closest confidants. Even in cases of severe mental illness, such as bipolar disorder, adhering strictly to a sleep and meal routine can lead to significant improvements.

The healing potential of micro-fasting is constantly growing as overeating and the number of meals and snacks per day increase, shortening the breaks between meals. The number of meals eaten per day has almost doubled since 1980, from three to around five or six on average. This new practice is instilled in children from an early age. After breakfast, the average school-age child eats a mid-morning snack, then lunch, then an afternoon snack, then dinner, another snack at half-time during a game of football and then perhaps another snack before going to bed. In Switzerland, the snack times between meals are known as 'Znüni' (the nine-o'clock meal) and 'Zvieri' (the four-o'clock meal). Linguistically speaking, this places them on an equal footing with the standard mealtimes 'Zmorge' (the morning meal), 'Zmittag' (the midday meal) and 'Znacht' (the evening meal). They carry the explicit instruction to parents, school staff and employers to plan enough time for a snack at 9 a.m. and 4 p.m. For children who have grown up with this practice, a fasting period of even three hours is a real challenge. An American woman who moved to France with her family told me how shocked she was by the French tradition of weaning young people off snacks – except for fruit in the afternoon. After resisting it for a while, however, she gave up and explained to her children that going hungry and feeling hungry were not the same thing. Soon she was even enthusiastic about withdrawing snacks: at mealtimes, her children ate happily and enjoyed their meals more and they were also mentally fitter, as reflected in better school performance.

Some of the health advantages of micro-fasting stem from the quality of foods, because a higher number of meals is often associated with increased consumption of processed fast food. After all, who has the time to prepare a fresh meal six times a day? By the same token, reducing the number of meals per day can improve the quality of those meals, since main meals are almost always healthier than snacks.

Methods of macro-fasting

Medically speaking, fasting is typically defined as complete or partial abstinence from certain foods, drinks and stimulants for a specific period of time, usually one or more days. Classical fasting, also known as therapeutic fasting, typically lasts seven to ten days and can be undertaken once or twice a year. Fore-going a specific kind of food or stimulant or limiting consumption of these is known as abstinence. Emptying the body reduces hunger and is consistent with the spiritual notion of cleansing. Depending on the chosen method, drinks and small quantities of food may be recommended to make fasting more pleasant. In the case of Buchinger fasting, which is particularly popular in Germany, adherents begin by voiding their bowels using Glauber's salt and enemas. This is followed by a process of 'setting up' with small quantities of fruit, rice, fresh food and water. This form of fasting does not require you to be an expert at starving yourself because calories are permitted; in fact, it promotes a transition to healthy eating with whole, plant-based foods (more on this in the next chapter). Other methods of fasting involve drinking raw juices, whey and herbal teas. These are thought to promote detoxification and skin health, but they have the disadvantage of causing blood sugar spikes that sharpen hunger pangs. In the Mayr method, adherents undergo a purge before being permitted to drink milk and mindfully chew bread rolls. The advantages of this are that milk is a complete food and bread is a source of carbohydrate, but doesn't cause sugar spikes. The downside is that milk and bread rolls are hardly particularly inspiring and do not set a good example of a healthy diet once the fast is complete.

Intermittent fasting is a surprisingly effective weight-loss strategy that requires fasters to extend their natural nighttime fasts regularly. The 16:8 method sees fasters leave sixteen hours between the last meal of the day and the first meal of the following day. Two meals can then be eaten during the following eight-hour window. The 14:10 method cuts fasting time to fourteen hours. The 12:12 method corresponds to the usual rhythm, with three meals a day, though this is becoming a challenge for increasing numbers of people because they have never done without the snacks between meals they enjoyed in childhood. In the 5:2 method, people eat normally for five days of the week and fast for two. The fasting days ought not to be consecutive. In alternate-day fasting, also known as the 1:1 method, people eat normally on one day, then fast the next, limiting their calorie intake to no more than a quarter of their regular intake.

Fasting at intervals allows the body to tap into its various energy reserves, thanks to a dip in insulin levels. The speed at which the following steps occur varies according to a person's constitution and nutrition. The first to be consumed is sugar, which is stored in the liver as glycogen. The body then begins to use its fat stores for energy. A consequence of this is that there is so little sugar remaining in the body that the metabolism creates ketones out of fat tissue, which serve as a sugar substitute for the brain. The depletion of fat reserves is healthy, as these reserves can cause metabolic issues, such as inflammation. Why would you attach a huge petrol tank to the roof of your car if there were a petrol station every sixty miles or so? The tank would not extend the car's lifespan; it would shorten it, placing a burden on the engine, transmission and wheels. There is also a chance it will rust and dirty the car. Incidentally, it is not true that fasting burns muscle, which you sometimes hear. Fasting specifically targets and metabolises fat, not muscle mass. Muscle mass begins to be depleted only when the body's fat percentage drops below five per cent, which is why people who are underweight are encouraged to avoid macro-fasting. In people who are of normal weight or overweight, fasting can even support muscle development, because meals and snacks can suppress the release of growth hormones by up to eighty per cent. Consequently, fasting is a powerful and natural trigger for releasing the growth hormones that promote muscle and bone development. Our ancestors benefited greatly from this effect, though involuntarily, due to a lack of food. But why should we forego its potential benefits?

The rapid weight loss that can occur during fasting is usually due to water loss, which lowers blood pressure and reduces the burden on the heart and blood vessels. Water loss results from low insulin levels, which signal the body to relax and detox. Water loss also results in a loss of potassium, calcium, magnesium and phosphorus, but the body can draw on its enormous mineral reserves in the bones to replace them. Fasting is also a very effective way to calm the sugar and insulin system sustainably. Regular consumption of sugar in fast food leads to mutually-reinforcing blood sugar and insulin spikes. This phenomenon is known as the glycaemic roller coaster. It may increase the risk of a host of health issues, such as headaches, migraine, depression, dementia, arterial calcification, kidney and eye conditions and certain cancers.[1] Among the known reasons for this are saccharification of the blood vessels and the release of free radicals due to oxidative stress. Oxidative stress occurs when the balance between the production of free radicals, which are chemically aggressive and the body's ability to neutralise them with antioxidants, is disrupted. Free radicals can cause genetic damage and can promote cancer when combined with insulin spikes, which serve as growth signals.

Fasting reduces inflammatory responses and has a positive impact on autoimmune diseases by lowering insulin levels and activating the vagus nerve. The effects this exhibits on the immune system are even more radical in people who are overweight because immune cells originate in fat tissue or, more accurately, in the thymus behind the breastbone and in bone marrow. They will happily wander into excess fatty tissue because they feel at home there. This can lead to the body being overpopulated with immune cells, raising the risk of autoimmune diseases and severe infections. Reducing fatty tissue through diet restriction and fasting can restore balance to the immune system. In this context, we often refer to starving out inflammation cells.[2]

The positive effects of fasting on the brain have also been documented in animals. Autophagy is the term given to the natural process of breaking down and recycling damaged or dead cell components in the brain. This method of waste disposal keeps the brain young. The reduction in blood sugar, insulin and inflammatory processes also protects the brain against neurodegenerative diseases such as dementia. Fasting also improves neuroplasticity, our mental 'openness' and capacity for learning and increases the distribution of noradrenaline, the neurotransmitter responsible for alertness. The ketone bodies that form during fasting calm the brain and protect it against overexcitation. They can also induce a mild euphoria, making fasting easier. This matches the experiences of people who report that fasting helps them achieve a more open, transparent and calmer mind, positive thoughts and a greater capacity for meditation. All these processes can be activated by a period of fasting for just six hours and increase considerably in the first twenty-four hours. Increased neuroplasticity could be one reason fasting has been adopted as a spiritual practice worldwide. The Ancient Greeks, for instance, were convinced that they could solve problems and puzzles more effectively while fasting.

The Norwegian writer and winner of the Nobel Prize for Literature, Knut Hamsun, captures the mental effects of ketone bodies and neuroplasticity in striking terms. As a young man, Hamsun was walking the streets of Oslo, looking for somewhere to eat:

> I had remarked so plainly that, whenever I had been hungry for any length of time, it was just as if my brains ran quite gently out of my head and left me with a vacuum – my head grew light and far off, I no longer felt its weight on my shoulders […] I was drunk with starvation; my hunger had made me tipsy. […] I had no pain – my hunger had taken the edge off it. In its stead, I felt pleasantly empty, untouched by everything around me, and glad not to be noticed by anyone. I put my feet up on the seat and leaned back. Thus, I could best appreciate the well-being of perfect isolation. There was not a cloud on my mind, not a feeling of discomfort, and, so far as my thought reached, I had not a whim, not a desire unsatisfied. I lay with open eyes, in a state of utter absence of mind. I felt myself charmed away. […] I entered into the joyous frenzy of hunger. I was empty and free from pain, and I gave free rein to my thoughts. In all calmness, I turn things over in my mind. […] …I did not even feel hunger so badly as some hours previously. I could hold out well till the next day.[3]

Hamsun's experience suggests that fasting not only keeps us physically fit but also mentally fit. Fasting increases resilience by mimicking famine, just as saunas replicate the effects of a heatwave and swimming in a cold lake can pre-empt and help our bodies practice for a cold snap. Abstinence and resisting temptation are essential elements of self-control. Small successes in fasting, such as foregoing bread at breakfast, can develop into bigger ones, such as avoiding snacks between meals. People who can withstand hunger pangs may also find it easier to let feelings of envy, jealousy, hatred, resentment and a desire for revenge pass by without reacting. In Aboriginal communities, forgoing food always retains an element of self-sacrifice, tied to the view that you occasionally have to give something up to improve your mental health.

Of course, fasting, like any effective treatment, can also have side effects. These include tiredness, exhaustion, headaches and low mood. It is not yet clear how swiftly, at what frequency and to what extent the positive effects occur, or how long they last. What we do know, however, is that intermittent fasting is an appropriate method for breaking down fat deposits and protecting blood vessels against saccharification. These are quick-onset health benefits which are easy to measure. Similarly, fasting has also been shown to have a positive impact on diabetes, gout and inflammation. Patients with these conditions should, however, only fast under their doctor's supervision. People who suffer from reflux – irritation in the lower part of the oesophagus – should not undertake periods of fasting without medical supervision because it can lead to a temporary increase in stomach acid. Feeling hungry while fasting is normal, but nausea, feeling unwell, dizziness, vomiting and weakness are not. If these symptoms persist for several hours, stopping is advised.

Fasting as a liminal experience

Fasting as a form of conscious abstinence has existed for around eight thousand years, since the advent of agriculture led to an abundance of food. Before this, intermittent fasting was a regular part of life, along with missing meals and going days without food. Hunter-gatherers were not always lucky when it came to finding food and the food that they did find could not be stored. Drought, conflict and insect infestations also led to more extended periods of hunger. The human body adapted to food shortages, which may explain why fasting is so good for us: it mimics the situation that our bodies were familiar with for thousands of years and to which they were best adjusted. As periods of involuntary hunger lessened, spiritual leaders were quick to recognise that constant, chaotic eating offered no advantage to either body or mind. They most likely observed an increase in previously unseen illnesses and concluded that certain foods or certain eating practices were polluting the body.

Fasting is the oldest known spiritual practice. The Ayurveda considers contamination through food to be the leading cause of all physical and mental illnesses and recommends purifying, detoxifying and cleansing body and mind through voluntary fasting. It also views fasting as a means for preventing illness and improving well-being.

The Buddha explored the limits of his capacity

for fasting on his road to enlightenment. Born into a wealthy family, he left his parents' house as a young man to seek enlightenment as an abstainer. One of the steps he took was to follow an extreme diet suggested to him by another wandering abstainer. He adhered strictly to the diet and lost weight and was soon so thin and lanky that a young woman named Sujata took pity on him and offered him some milk-rice pudding, which he took as an opportunity to break his fast. He felt that the food did him good and did not disturb his meditation but instead deepened it, giving him the strength to sit under the bodhi tree and experience a spiritual awakening. He had to admit that the ascetic diet had been a dead-end for him. Admittedly, it had helped him to lose weight temporarily and to suppress his needs, but it had not supported his well-being or his spiritual awakening. His meditation on this experience of existential boundary-testing and human suffering led him to teach the Middle Way, a midpoint between indulgence and ascetic torment that leads to a higher and freer existence. Until the end of his life, he maintained a focus on the right way to address hunger and the social and ecological impacts of food. This gave rise to his command not to reject food which is offered to you, an expression of his deep gratitude for life. In an impressive example of this belief in action, the Buddha once ate a poisoned dish out of respect for his host. The food in question varies according to the telling, but it is thought to have been either spoiled pork or poisonous mushrooms that led the Buddha to fall ill and enter

Nirvana. As varied as the stories of his passing are, all of them see him having the taste of umami on his tongue as he closed his eyes for the last time.

The limits to fasting, which the Buddha explored, are known in medicine as metabolic flexibility. This refers to the ability to switch quickly between fat formation and fat breakdown. People can learn this ability much like a language by eating on a regular schedule and avoiding snacks. However, some people have limited metabolic flexibility. These include people with eating disorders (such as bulimia), people with a slim build, children under eighteen, pregnant women and nursing mothers, none of whom should fast for longer than twelve hours at a time.

Fasting as a spiritual reset

A spiritual reset is the process or practice of distancing oneself from daily distractions, negative energies, or habits to achieve a deeper connection with oneself, the universe, or a higher self. Much like a physical reset where a device or system is returned to its original settings, a spiritual reset means liberating oneself from emotional, mental, or spiritual blocks.

Fasting is the oldest and most widespread method of achieving a reset of this kind, through cleansing, refreshment, rejuvenation and connection. The origins of this practice are most likely to be found in our ancestors' belief that demonic forces could be imbibed through food and drink. Fasting offered surefire protection against such forces. The lighter and purer the dish, the softer and purer the soul. This idea experienced a boom alongside the notion that fasting actively drives evil spirits out of the body. This belief lives on in the Christian tradition of preparing one's soul for Easter with a purifying fast. The next boost to this practice saw people using ascetic fasting to focus their mental energy, with a view to achieving ecstasy or ascending to higher spiritual spheres. The Desert Fathers and John the Baptist fasted in solitude to increase their spiritual hunger and prepare themselves for transcendental revelations. Even Jesus had to undergo a forty-day fast to prove his godly calling. Reduced forms of fasting facilitated mental and physical processes of transformation in everyday life. Fasting rites served to stimulate fertility and prepared young people undergoing puberty for acceptance into adult society. Fasting after a bereavement helped those left behind to process the death of their loved one.

Scholars were among the first to discover that a metabolic reset – aimed at optimising and recalibrating the body's metabolism – helped improve health and rid people of bad habits. Fasting can calm the inflammatory and digestive systems and this was considered a good prerequisite for a mental clean slate. Teaching in the early Middle Ages, the Christian monk and influential ascetic John Climacus wrote: 'Leather bottles get greater capacity if they are supple, but if they are left in neglect, they do not hold so much. He who burdens his stomach with food, distends his inside; but he who wars with his stomach contracts it. And when the inside is contracted, then we cannot take much and in the future, we become faster naturally.' According to John, the soul also benefits from this regeneration of the gut:

'Fasting is the coercion of nature and the cutting out of everything that delights the palate, the prevention of lust, the uprooting of bad thoughts, deliverance from dreams, purity of prayer, the light of the soul, the guarding of the mind, deliverance from blindness, the door of compunction, humble sighing, glad contrition, a lull in chatter, a means to silence, a guard of obedience, lightening of sleep, health of body, agent of dispassion, remission of sins, the gate of Paradise and its delight.'[4]

Fasting may have physical benefits, but it can also help people learn their limits and let go of bad habits, negative energy and thoughts. It can also strengthen psychological resilience by fostering processes of mental change, particularly after a loss, during separation and grief and at the beginning of a new project or chapter of life. Ultimately, fasting is a simple and effective practice of contentment, offering enormous potential for happiness because it enables us to look at the world anew and see it as rewarding and satisfying.

Fasting in animals and humans

Some animals fast for days or even months at a time and a few of them fast or sleep through the winter. This typically occurs due to a lack of food and to avoid the dangers of hunting. Crocodiles, snakes, frogs, dragonflies, aardvarks, lemurs, snails, lungfish and crabs can fast for several months without incurring harm. This habit can be observed in frogs, which fast over winter and are then able to jump as high in spring as they would in winter because their period of fasting protects their muscles against metabolic autophagy. By contrast, other animals, such as mice and rats, are incapable of fasting. The longer they go without food, the more nervous and restless they become. Humans, however, are among those lifeforms which are capable of fasting. The ability to fast was one of the prerequisites for leaving the tropics and inhabiting regions where parts of the year are inhospitable and food supplies are unreliable. It is no coincidence that traditional periods of fasting tend to fall at the end of winter when, in the past, food stores would have gradually run low.

It is not just our bodies that are designed for these kinds of shortages; our minds are too. We know this because human beings find it almost impossible to imagine an abundance of food. It makes it exceptionally easy for the food industry to trick us into believing that food is scarce. If nothing else, we have learned that excessive salt and calories are not good for us, even though both are essential nutritional components that our bodies cannot produce themselves. We have learned from experiences in food processing and many foods now contain more nutrients than they did just after the Second World War. Flour is less white than it was thirty years ago because it is now refined less, removing less of the fibre and rice contains more micronutrients than it did during our grandparents' time. Fertilisers and animal feed also contain increasingly high levels of essential micronutrients, such as vitamins, copper, selenium and zinc, which are reflected in higher levels of these nutrients in our food.

This increase in micronutrient intake may lead to an increased risk of hypervitaminosis. This is a condition caused by abnormally high vitamin doses and is usually attributed to high-dose supplements. The most dangerous are the liposoluble vitamins A, D and E. A high intake of these vitamins can manifest with symptoms of poisoning, such as headaches, weakness, dizziness, nausea, constipation, diarrhoea, internal tremors and an inability to engage in physical activity or carry out one's daily routine. A dose of just 120 IU (international units a day, which is lower than the dosage of certain freely available vitamin E supplements, may increase the risk of brain haemorrhage.[5]

Managing hunger

Given the many benefits of fasting, I'm pretty surprised I didn't take it up sooner. A subconscious fear of hunger was probably what prompted my initial scepticism.

Fortunately, any fears I had were exaggerated, as I learned while losing weight after several years of living in the US. Our ability to fast includes various mechanisms that alleviate hunger from the day after the beginning of the fast. Fasting would never have become so popular if this were not the case. This phenomenon can be explained physiologically by a drop in insulin levels around ten hours in, which helps keep hunger under control. After one day, the stomach also begins to produce less of the hunger hormone ghrelin, which leads to a greater sense of relaxation. After a few days, the gut hormones leptin and ghrelin, which are responsible for acute hunger, hand over the reins to some extent and other hormones – those responsible for long-term survival and metabolism, such as agouti-related protein - take over. This makes sense from an evolutionary perspective because severe hunger pangs during natural periods of starvation could have led us to eat harmful or dangerous foods out of desperation. Instead, these hormones consider the long term and do not react to exaggerated fears of starvation; they are aware of the fundamental truth that empty stores are better than full ones, because storing unnecessary nutrients is costly and can cause inflammation, as can be observed in people who are overweight. Every additional kilogram of fat causes inflammation to spread further through the body.[6] Tests on yeasts, worms, rodents and apes demonstrate that this inflammation impairs metabolism and tissue regeneration.[7] A constant supply of food accelerates the ageing process, while food restrictions and empty stores are, as yet, the best-known anti-ageing methods and can increase life expectancy by up to thirty per cent.

There is practical significance to the hunger-suppressing effects of intermittent fasting, i.e. changing one's eating patterns by missing the same meal every day. We can observe this mechanism in ourselves without intermittent fasting by fasting overnight. Sensations of hunger are typically minimal just after getting up, even though we have not eaten all night. This mechanism is used in a targeted way in intermittent fasting. Skipping a meal may require a lot of effort initially, but our bodies soon adapt to the new rhythm and our hunger disappears. You only notice that this requires a specific kind of self-control when you slip up and break your intermittent fast. This typically leads to feelings of ferocious hunger at the same time the next day, because we can train ourselves not just to feel satisfied, but also to feel hungry. If we're used to eating a hearty breakfast in the mornings, we will feel appropriately hungry when we wake up. Yet this does not reflect a physiological need; it is simply an expression of the hunger patterns to which we have grown accustomed. The Hadza, a nomadic hunter-gatherer people in East Africa, remind us that breakfast is a modern invention. They do not eat right away when they get up because there is no food available to them. By late morning, they will eat freshly gathered berries. This equates to a fasting period of ten to fourteen hours. Of course, I don't mean to suggest that skipping breakfast is the best option. The time we choose to forego a meal is not the decisive factor and our bodies can adjust to different fasting patterns.

Many other mental schedules govern hunger and have almost nothing to do with calorie requirements, aside from sleep, diurnal rhythm and the regularity of food consumption. Even if we're not feeling especially peckish, the aroma of a grilled steak and the sound of sizzling can make us feel hungry. Many of these stimuli are innate and others we learn in childhood or later in life.

The Russian psychologist Ivan Pavlov received the

Nobel Prize for his research into how hunger is learned by experimenting on dogs. As part of his research, he took to measuring the dogs' saliva. Whenever he fed the dogs, they would salivate more, thereby proving that food stimulates appetite. This is an important finding and explains why we ought not to leave snacks lying around our workplaces or homes. Yet this insight alone was not enough to win Pavlov the Nobel Prize. He also observed that the dogs' saliva levels increased even when he approached their cage without food. The dogs had learned that the sound of Pavlov's footsteps meant food was on its way. The sound of his footsteps was enough to trigger the hunger process. This is known as conditioning, in which the meaning of food becomes a stimulus unrelated to the food itself. In later experiments, Pavlov resorted to ringing a bell, which did not initially prompt an increase in saliva production. However, when he continued ringing the bell after the dogs were fed, they began to salivate whenever it rang, even if food never materialised. Our appetites are conditioned in the same way, typically to specific times of day. This makes sense, provided this conditioning is appropriate for our calorific needs. It ensures we eat regularly, which is good for us, because our conditioning prepares our bodies to take in food.

Fasting requires adjustments to our usual temporal conditioning, but fortunately, these typically occur within a few days. When fasting, it is important to avoid conditioning triggers such as the sound of a cornflakes packet or the smell drifting from bakeries or restaurants, because, much like Pavlov's bell, they will trigger the appetite. Alongside these typical conditionings, which we are all subject to, every individual should be aware of their own triggers. It could be television, being in the car, a particular film or a song. The more able we are to resist these triggers and only eat at the dinner table at designated times, the quicker they will lose their impact. This was another of Pavlov's discoveries: the longer he left the bell to ring when there was no food, the less the dogs reacted to the sound. This is known as deconditioning or unlearning. When it comes to un-learning triggers, it can be helpful to replace eating with another activity, such as drinking tea or black coffee. This method lessens withdrawal symptoms. Exercise is a particularly effective way to unlearn hunger triggers be-cause anaerobic respiration produces lactic acid, which actively reduces appetite. Burning calories can reduce hunger and avoiding snacks between meals, or even whole meals, can stimulate our desire to exercise. This might seem illogical at first, but our metabolism does not operate with a bookkeeper's logic; it operates *psycho-logically*, in pursuit of self-efficacy. The more we exercise and reduce calorie intake, the more pleasure we take in it. By contrast, artificial sweeteners are poorly positioned to reduce hunger because they stimulate insulin release, thereby increasing physiological hunger. Keeping busy is one promising strategy in the face of this. When we spend time we would usually be eating working instead. It is easy to withstand the wave of conditioned hunger without relapsing.

Alongside hunger, which is often triggered unnecessarily for the reasons described above, we also face the issue of being unable to rely on our feelings of satiety. It is indicative of a more fundamental problem: we are neither physically nor mentally prepared for excess. When our ancestors arrived in a place filled with fruit and animals, finding, preparing and chewing healthy food naturally entailed great effort and risk. As a result, they had to ask themselves whether they were truly hungry. The unconscious, perpetual hunger that we experience today would not have developed in these kinds of circumstances. This is why our natural sense of satiety never says, 'On no account should you eat that hamburger, you're full!' Consciously foregoing food that is available to us ready-made is a new problem that must be dealt with actively and consciously.

Fasting is one solution to this problem and, in every culture, it is bound up with morality. What constituted morality was once a fear of God and the need to cleanse oneself spiritually. Today, the emphasis tends to be placed on health. Modern moralising will say, 'You ought not to eat that, it's unhealthy, it'll make you fat and you'll end up with Type 2 diabetes.' Social anxieties will then follow this: 'Do you really think no one's noticed that huge pile of chips on your plate? Aren't you embarrassed?' Yet there is also an opposing moralising voice known as the obscene superego. The superego says, 'You've got to eat it! You love this food – stand up for what you want!' The basic aim of all moralising voices is freedom in a comprehensive sense: freedom from hunger and from shame. However, the obscene voice confuses this all-encompassing freedom with fleeting feelings of freedom and arbitrariness – it pays too little attention to the fact that long-term freedom requires limitations in the moment. Consequently, fasting is a good opportunity to become aware of your moral compass and deeper desires. Does my notion of freedom involve eating however many doughnuts I want in one hour, or does it entail still being able to go on trips with my friends, grandchildren, or godchildren when I'm in my seventies? Freedom is the fundamental difference between starving and fasting: starving is foregoing food involuntarily. People who are starving do not know when they will eat their next meal. By contrast, fasting is voluntarily abstaining from food for health, spiritual, or other reasons. A desire for freedom is typically what drives many people's fascination with fasting. In extreme cases, hunger strikes are employed to achieve greater independence. Mahatma Gandhi successfully undertook a campaign of fasting to protest against British colonial rule in India.

A practical approach

When planning a fast, the following question often arises: What should I do if I feel hungry or unwell? What if I can't stand it? What if I don't feel like myself anymore? What if I go mad with hunger and start smashing plates? The answer is simple, however: eat something!

If you feel unable to fast, consider the points below.

Unnecessarily high expectations and being too quick to adjust your eating patterns are among the key reasons why people abandon fasting. If you regularly eat snacks between meals, you're better off starting with micro-fasting, which aims to forgo snacks and focus on main meals. To prepare your body for fasting, these meals should be eaten at the same time every day. One of the most significant findings from my own research was that spending too little or irregular time in bed increases appetite, as it disrupts our sleep-wake cycle.[8] I say time in bed, not time asleep, because lying down peacefully in bed from 10 p.m. to 6 a.m. is enough to get into a good rhythm. Sleep is all well and good, but in this case, it's not required to regulate our appetites.

Alongside unrealistic expectations and disrupted rhythms, eating the wrong food can also cause us to fail in our attempts at fasting. Processed sugars and a lack of fruits and vegetables, which contain natural proteins and complex carbohydrates, can leave us with unbearably keen appetites. A lack of adequate hydration and a massive increase in sports and exercise can also contribute to this problem. Emotional eating is another key obstacle on the path to a satisfying fast. In this case, hunger is not an expression of physical need or a metabolic function; instead, it helps process stress and regulate feelings. Emotional hunger typically arises on a whim, triggered by thoughts and feelings. By contrast, physical hunger develops more slowly and begins with a rumble in your stomach. Only certain foodstuffs can satisfy emotional hunger, such as cream cakes or chocolates. In contrast, physical hunger will respond to any calories, even those found in foods you might not like. Emotional hunger can grow into episodes of all-out binge eating, while physical hunger will disappear after eating a regular portion of food. Emotional eating also often leads to feelings of shame, regret and guilt, which rarely occur when we sate our physical hunger. Emotional eating also includes the aforementioned misconception that you are suffering from a nutrient deficiency, which, realistically, can be put down to dubious advertising, industry-sponsored reporting and pseudoscientific blood tests.

Recognising that hunger is not a simple, rational cue but more akin to an insatiable desire with higher aims beyond simply taking in calories is ancient wisdom. Feelings of hunger are at the centre of how Buddhism views suffering. According to Buddhist psychology, hunger comprises two different 'pillars': an immediate, physical sensation and a reaction to this sensation which is bound up with emotions such as desire, unease, or aversion, as well as thoughts like 'I have to eat something urgently!' Buddhist mindfulness aims to help decouple this immediate, physical sensation of hunger from the emotional, mental reaction to it: 'Yes, there is hunger in my body', a Buddhist teacher once replied to me, smiling, without making the slightest move towards responding to it.

The Buddha did not concern himself only with the psychological and spiritual aspects of hunger; he was also aware that social factors play a crucial role in fasting.

Fasting in a group, such as in a monastery, is easier than fasting alone. Solitary fasts undertaken for health, psychological, or spiritual reasons often fail due to social pressure. Rejecting an invitation to a communal meal has always been a serious matter. It leaves many people feeling upset or personally attacked. As I will explain in a later chapter on communal eating, this reaction is understandable and is deeply rooted in our history. We must take the interpersonal functions of communal eating very seriously and adjust our fasting to the circumstances, so as not to provoke any negative social consequences. Thus, it is important to interrupt one's fast for special occasions such as birthdays or weddings. But before I go deeper into communal eating and eating rituals, let's take a look at the next chapter, which focuses on the foods on which our bodies depend.

Whole Foods

The American journalist, Michael Pollan, summarises his years of investigative work and his thinking about healthy eating in three short sentences: 'Eat food. Not too much. Mostly plants.'[1] The latter two sentences are not particularly surprising, but the first one gives me pause: realistically, the foods we eat ought to be 'whole' foods, such as a whole apple or whole beans.

To further understand Michael Pollan's view, I will need to look backwards a little and expand on the ideas that I mentioned in the introduction. According to current nutritional theory, food is composed of macro- and micronutrients and the composition and balance of these nutrients determine how healthy a food is. It makes no difference, this theory claims, whether nutrients come from a tablet or from a whole apple. When I was studying medicine, I learned this theory too, so I was astonished to learn that practical medicine deviated from it with surprising consistency. While training in internal medicine, I saw nurses disconnect a patient from her feeding tube and invite her to feed herself. Even though the tube-fed supplements provided a much richer, more balanced supply of nutrients, the chief physician insisted that bread rolls, yoghurt and gruel were the healthier option. To me, this behaviour seemed old-fashioned. It seemed like the kind of wisdom you would pick up from your grandmother, insisting that eating natural foods was inherently beneficial. As an assistant physician at the Eating Disorders Centre at the University of Zurich, I was confronted once again with the apparently widespread medical imperative to promote whole foods. My superior asked me to remove the liquid foods my patients liked and to help them get used to solid foods. I did this begrudgingly because I could not see any scientific justification for why solid food could be more beneficial than liquid food. This change in diet undoubtedly led to a distinct reduction in the balanced nature and nutritional content of the food consumed by patients who, due to their eating disorders, tended to have strong aversions to whole foods and ate a much less varied diet in the absence of liquid food. Fortunately, my superior was not only an experienced general practitioner but also well-versed in the scientific literature. Using observational studies, she showed me that liquid foods increased the risk of exhaustion, digestive complaints, metabolic issues (including sugar metabolism) and osteoporosis, even though they contained considerably more nutrients than solid foods. She didn't know why, but what is and remains clear is that clinical experience contradicts the nutritional theory as presented in some textbooks.

The most unmistakable evidence for Pollan's call to eat whole foods is seen in patients who cannot eat normally due to medical conditions, such as bowel paralysis and must be fed parenterally. The 'par' here means 'next to', while 'enteral' essentially refers to the gut; together they describe a process of bypassing the bowel, be it via injection or an intravenous infusion. These nutrient solutions contain a perfect blend of macro and micronutrients – enough to send any food chemist into raptures. They include all the necessary vitamins (including thiamine, ascorbic acid, niacin, riboflavin and biotin), all essential amino acids (including methionine, phenylalanine and tryptophan), all essential fatty acids (including Omega-3 fatty acids) and all the essential trace elements (including zinc, selenium, magnesium, calcium, iron, sodium, potassium, phosphorus, copper and iodine), as well as creatine, folic acid, carbohydrates, protein and fat, all of which are measured out to the nearest milligram according to the standards set by international guidelines. Experienced doctors will only use parenteral feeding as a last resort when all other feeding options have failed.

Another example of whole foods in action is fruit juice. Even though fruit juices have the same chemical composition as whole fruits, they are comparatively less healthy due to their lower fibre content compared to their whole fruit counterpart. Whole fruits, by contrast, are more nutritious and consuming fruit in its whole food matrix can lower the risk of non-communicable diseases.

Is depression a nutrient deficiency?

Theories of nutrient deficiencies are increasingly influencing my own field: psychiatry. Over the course of my own research, my doubts about these theories grew. I caught the first hints of unspoken issues with nutritional studies in 2003, when I embarked on three years of research at the National Institute of Mental Health, the USA's state institute for psychiatric research. At the time, one cause of depression was believed to be an absence of the neurotransmitter and happiness hormone, serotonin. The amino acid tryptophan is the chemical precursor to serotonin, so there was discussion as to whether a tryptophan deficiency could explain depression. When I suggested to the director of the department for research into depression that we look more closely into the serotonin-deficiency theory, he refused: 'We've carried out dozens of studies into this theory and I can assure you that people with depression do not suffer from a serotonin-deficiency. We've investigated brain tissue using imaging procedures, as well as genetics. There is no indication that these people suffer from a lack of serotonin. If you put healthy people on a diet rich in amino acids but lacking tryptophan, over time, a distinct tryptophan deficiency develops in the brain, leading to a deficiency of serotonin. But the subjects tested showed no sign of depression. We also gave depressive patients tryptophan, but they only grew more depressed. This theory stinks and we've decided to stop working on it.'

I was flabbergasted and asked him why, in that case, antidepressants did not increase serotonin levels in the brain. He replied, 'We know very little about the effects of antidepressants. What we do know is that they inhibit the reuptake of serotonin in nerve cells, meaning that serotonin cannot be recycled. This may lead to a short-term rise in serotonin in the synapses, but after a couple of weeks, it drops again and it is at that point that antidepressants truly begin to take effect.' I had come well prepared and reminded him that he had himself written articles on serotonin deficiency. He replied, saying, 'I do believe that serotonin has a role to play in depression, but not due to a deficiency. I prefer the term serotonin dysfunction. But you're probably right, the serotonin deficiency theory is so popular that people occasionally use the term 'serotonin deficiency' to express the fact that depression has something to do with the brain. We have lots of jobs to do as doctors, so we must develop theories that our patients can actually understand. The industry also needs theories of deficiencies. Everyone understands that companies manufacture chemicals to treat chemical deficiencies. No one would understand a company producing chemicals to treat an excess of certain chemicals in the body But don't get me wrong, antidepressants are an effective treatment, even if the serotonin-deficiency theory has proved untrue.'

I found this conversation exciting, but it left me feeling uneasy. Still, it was this experience that gave me my first inkling that there are various realities in medicine. It brought to mind the ruptures in the scientific worldview that had captured my interest since childhood. In Lucerne, where I grew up, the water contains high levels of calcium and magnesium, requiring regular descaling of household appliances.

Even so, health magazines in the region still warn of a calcium and magnesium deficiency that up to fifty per cent of the population is supposed to be suffering from – something that certainly cannot be true in Lucerne. On one occasion, a pharmacist came to visit and I asked him why he had calcium and magnesium tablets in his shop window. He laughed, replying, 'Those are for the Italian tourists. We don't need them.'

But back to Pollan's view on food. It implies not just that the wholeness of foods is more important than their micronutrient composition. Still, wholeness is more important than the balance of macronutrients such as carbohydrates, fats and proteins. Nutrient solutions are much better at maintaining a balance of these kinds of nutrients than natural foods are. What is interesting, however, is that people in the Blue Zones – where people take pleasure in food and live longer lives – predominantly eat whole foods and don't care a jot for the balance of nutrients recommended by modern food chemistry. For example, people living along the Mediterranean consume far more fatty foods than is recommended. The fat content of the food they eat amounts to almost fifty per cent. By the same token, people living longer lives in Central America primarily eat maize and beans, meaning that carbohydrates make up seventy-five per cent of their diets. And the diet enjoyed by the Masai in East Africa – a people almost untouched by the diseases of modern society – is very high in protein – over fifty per cent – because they predominantly consume cow's blood, meat and milk.

These findings must lead us to conclude that the chemical-focused concept of nutrition fails even when it comes to the critical factor of balance. Even randomised studies in which participants were divided into different dietary groups, each consuming different levels of carbohydrate, fat and protein, never proved that a specific macronutrient composition conferred health benefits.[2] Similarly, the idea that macronutrients are important for health does not stem from university research laboratories; it was invented by industry. The food industry can change the fat, carbohydrate and protein content of the foodstuffs it produces at will. All theories of chemical nutrition typically express the same message: processed foods and dietary supplements can provide the same health benefits as whole, natural foods which have not been chemically manipulated.

I'm keen to emphasise the blind spots in the theory of chemical nutrition because it has asserted itself worldwide in the media since the 1980s, is increasingly enshrined in law and is taught in schools. What it has not done, however, is improve public health; on the contrary, it is the very heart of the problem and has led to a fourfold increase in cases of Type 2 diabetes, a doubling in rates of obesity and a considerable rise in autoimmune diseases. Just take, for example, the Nutri-Score rating system, which has been keenly supported and advertised by big food companies since 2016. Scientists developed the Nutri-Score, which includes a few principles based on science, such as a positive rating for whole, unprocessed foods and it does not take into account added minerals and vitamins. The rating system runs from A (very healthy) to E (very unhealthy). In the current version of the system, chemical additives such as sweeteners, colouring agents and preservatives no longer equate to a lower rating. When the system was initially being developed, scientists set the quantity of added sugar deemed harmful at twenty-five grams per day. This was revised to ninety grams per day of total sugar, blurring the distinction between 'free' and 'added' sugar. It has also become increasingly possible to raise the score of completely unhealthy fast-food products by adding soluble fibre. A well-known Swiss chocolate milk brand I loved as a child now gets a B rating on the scale, meaning it is recommended for regular consumption – directly undermining my parents' insistence that I enjoy a glass only on special occasions. The logic is that milk is healthy and skimmed milk is even healthier. This is seen as justification for adding sugar for taste. However, every part of this argument is false: milk is only healthy for adults in small quantities and it may even be unhealthy for many people. The logic of the Nutri-Score system, which claims that removing fat from milk balances out the harmful effects of sugar, is entirely wrong. In fact, the opposite is true: both industrial measures serve only to increase the potentially damaging effects. The Nutri-Score system is based on a theory of food as an unconnected collection of units of nutritional value, which, rather than being the solution to the epidemic of diet-related illness witnessed in the 1980s, is what may have contributed to it in the first place. As the chocolate milk example demonstrates, illness and health cannot be explained, in large part, by individual nutrients, but rather by the interplay between nutrients, which is fundamentally different in whole foods than in highly processed foods.[3] These interactions also explain why parenteral feeding – which would be rated A for its perfect balance of nutrients – is so unhealthy. To sum up:

- What the industry's wishful thinking would have you think: the proportions of protein, carbohydrate and fat found in foods are crucial to their health-giving potential. The industry can reformulate these proportions at its discretion to make its foods comparable to natural foods.
- What the science says: studies have proven that the proportions of protein, carbohydrate and fat found in foods are surprisingly unimportant. When it comes to carbohydrates, what matters more is whether the carbohydrate is complex; for fats and proteins, variety seems to be most important. Compared to processed foods, natural foods contain a larger variety of proteins, more complex carbohydrates and more complex fats, which explains why they are beneficial to health.[4]

The food matrix

The food matrix refers to the crucial interplay of nutrients within a whole food. The lack of a food matrix may have contributed to Claudia's death, as I described in the introduction and this is why, as a young doctor, I was encouraged to replace my patients' liquid food with solid food. A matrix is a grid of sorts and, in this case, refers to the fact that the nutrients in a food are not dissolved in a liquid but are instead held together by complex biological structures – you might picture these as interwoven, three-dimensional grids. The external grid of a simple salad leaf is comprised of a protective waxy layer, an upper and lower epidermis, palisade cells, spongy tissue and stomata. The grid contains thousands of different antioxidants that protect the salad leaf. Within this grid, there are countless other grids. Plant cell walls are significant, forming an enclosed space that enables them to provide nutrients within a specific chemical environment. This sophisticated structure plays a decisive role in a food's nutritional value because it slows digestion, conserves nutrients that are quickly broken down, and ensures that the upper and lower bowel, as well as the entire microbiome, are well nourished. Onions are a good example of how foods undergo a complex transformation during digestion. Onions do not contain any nutrients that might irritate our eyes. The irritating substance in question does not form until the onion is cut; once its grid-like structure is destroyed, the nutrients begin to interact in new ways. A chemical reaction occurs between a sulphurous amino acid in the external grid and an enzyme which forms part of the internal grid. (Incidentally, freezing onions before cutting them prevents this chemical reaction from taking place.)

Our bodies have millions of years of experience with whole foods, leading us to develop a multi-stage digestive process in which the food matrix is broken down step by step. Each section of the bowel specialises in breaking down a particular grid and taking up the chemical compounds that arise during disintegration. An onion shows us that cutting through all the grids at once overwhelms our mucous membranes. In contrast, multi-stage digestive processes are constantly producing new nutrients that are suited to each respective section of the mucous membrane via the interaction between foodstuff and the bowel. The newly produced nutrients are often so ephemeral that it is impossible to identify them chemically. This may be a significant reason why perfect parenteral feeding solutions tend to lead to severe malnutrition: we still do not know many of the key nutrients that emerge during digestion and, due to their ephemeral nature, are unable to manufacture them in a non-perishable form. Producers of dietary supplements are required by law to indicate on the packaging of their products that dietary supplements are not a replacement for a varied diet.

Fibre is another important factor in the health-giving effects of whole foods:

- **What the industry suggests:** fibre can exhibit effects independent of the food matrix. There are soluble fibres which help to regulate blood sugar and blood lipids. There are also insoluble fibres which are not taken up by the digesta and travel through the gut unchanged, supporting digestion and feeding the gut bacteria. It is irrelevant whether these fibres are natural or industrially produced.
- **What the science says:** both facts about the

health-promoting aspects of fibre are correct, but that's only half the story. It is undoubtedly true that the extent of chemical cross-linking in a food plays a role. The foodstuffs with the most stable food matrices, such as fruits and vegetables, are also the healthiest because fibres bind the nutrients together in a great, three-dimensional grid, slowing down the uptake of nutrients and facilitating a multi-stage digestive process during which new nutrients emerge. This is why it is misguided to view fibre as a kind of vitamin that can be added to food. This is evident, for instance, in the fact that aboriginal peoples, such as the Hadza of Tanzania, demonstrate distinctly more diverse communities of gut bacteria than people living in the West, even though the latter add industrial fibre to their foods.[5]

The industry's beliefs are often shared by many consumers, including acquaintances and family members of mine. I occasionally get into debates with them about milk products and their alternatives and I tend to focus on almonds, among other things, in the hope of making a productive contribution to these kinds of discussions. Almonds are excellent natural products, boasting an exceptional matrix containing many fats and carbohydrates. It's why eating whole almonds will only cause a minimal rise in blood lipids. However, consuming powdered almonds, almond butter, or almond oil will prompt a considerably greater increase in blood lipids, even if the equivalent quantity of almonds is being consumed. Calorie intake is also noticeably higher in the latter case. Add to this the fact that we tend to eat far more powdered almonds, almond butter and almond oil at once than we do whole almonds, because there is no need to chew and our fullness cues respond less to oils and powders. This increases the harmful potential of processed almonds because almond sugar rises rapidly in the blood and can saccharify blood vessels.[6] I'm not trying to impose a ban on almond butter; I want to point out that ground and blended almonds have better health benefits if eaten slowly, mindfully and only in small quantities.

The banana is another impressive example of the food matrix in action. In its younger form, with pale green ends, almost all of a banana's carbohydrates are present as starch, which boasts a connective matrix. It passes through the stomach and small intestine almost undigested, then is broken down in the large intestine, much to the glee of any gut bacteria present. Digestion in the large intestine particularly strongly stimulates the vagus nerve.[7] By contrast, an overripe, brown banana contains just ten per cent of its former starch, with the rest having transformed into sugar. Its matrix is so weak that the small intestine absorbs it immediately, like fruit juice, prompting a less-than-advantageous flood of sugar into the bloodstream, activating the stress response and contributing to the malnourishment of gut flora.[8] A less ripe banana is also more filling than an overripe banana, because it slows digestion and in-hibits the release of insulin. New medications in the field of diabetes research, such as semaglutide, which is revolutionising the treatment of severe obesity and slow gastric emptying, which, in turn, slows digestion and reduces appetite. The same effect can be achieved much more cheaply and without side effects, by eating foods *al dente* with the matrix intact.[9] Due to a chemical reorganisation, cooling down foods such as rice, noodles and potatoes is a good way to enrich them with complex, resistant carbohydrates that slow digestion and serve as natural prebiotics, nourishing gut bacteria.

Unfortunately, the industry is currently unable to produce foods with a robust matrix. I feel particularly aware of this whenever I read about start-ups full of motivated young people inventing completely new foodstuffs by destroying the matrices of whole foods. I'm impressed by their desire to innovate and envision the world anew. Yet, it also gives me pause, because these kinds of new foods are contributing to the avalanche of obesity and Type 2 diabetes. If you want to manufacture a new foodstuff, you need emulsifiers, which hold nutrients together, because creating a matrix would be too expensive. However, this method is particularly harmful because emulsifiers are chemicals which act like detergents, rendering the everyday interactions between nutrients and the gut impossible. The result? A greater risk of obesity, Type 2 diabetes and disrupted gut bacteria.[10] Many trendy foods, such as celery crisps and gluten-free baked goods, contain emulsifiers and should therefore be enjoyed only in small amounts.

As any bodybuilder's body shape would suggest, it's not just plants that possess a complex, three-dimensional matrix; animals do too. Bundles of muscle fibres are held together by fascia and these bundles sit within connective tissue. A membrane surrounds every individual muscle fibre and contains numerous cells which are connected via connecting discs. Every individual muscle cell is its own cosmos, with a nucleus, energy-supplying mitochondria and various muscle proteins which form long chains. In highly processed meat, such as a hamburger patty, this matrix is severely damaged; the muscle is reduced to a puree, making it easier to eat and to avoid the healthy but occasionally strenuous digestive process. By contrast, inhabitants of the Blue Zones eat partially and fully raw meat with a crisp texture. Fish is particularly well-suited to this; it has a relatively weak matrix because it requires fewer muscle fibres to support its body in water.

How eating foods with intact food matrices can boost physical and mental stability

From my experience in the US, I learned that fast food not only contributes to weight gain, but it can also make you feel tired, like a gherkin with no sense of firmness or consistency. The latest research suggests that this sensation of feeling like a limp gherkin is not so far from the truth after all. One exciting study split foods into three groups. The unprocessed and minimally processed group included fruits, vegetables and rice, all of which have an intact food matrix – more of a firm cucumber than a limp gherkin. The processed foods included oils, butter, milk products and smoked meats – foods which have partially retained their matrix and probably fall under the same category as the gherkin. Listed under ultraprocessed foods were foodstuffs in which artificial substances such as emulsifiers, hydrogenated fats and other chemical additives were used to bind together naked calories loosely – these foods are more akin to cucumber juice, to stick with the original analogy. Scientists discovered that unconnected, empty calories were associated with a higher risk of anxiety, depressive symptoms and a reduction in mental faculties. At the same time, foods with an intact food matrix boosted resilience.[11] One possible explanation is that the limp gherkin and the cucumber juice are absorbed in the upper intestine, leaving gut flora malnourished and contributing to tiredness and exhaustion.

The industry purports to give its limp gherkins a boost with added vitamins. My father worked for a pharmaceutical company that manufactured vitamin C industrially. The studies the company carried out did not provide evidence of health benefits from added vitamin C. Even so, they spent millions of Swiss francs extolling the benefits of vitamin C to the world, even though their own studies did not provide this evidence. My father was shocked and disappointed and he chose to leave the company he had once admired for its commitment to scientific excellence. I'm not trying to say that there aren't people who depend on dietary supplements, be it due to digestive issues or eating disorders. Still, I want to stress that vitamins, calcium and fatty acid supplements are clear examples of foods that lack a matrix and offer the body little in the way of vigour. In nutritional supplements of this kind, nutrients are only present in molecules. The bad news about the harmful effects of vitamins and trace elements, which have been published in journals in recent years, relates to the chemical 'loneliness' of these nutrients. We have to assume that it's not just blood sugar spikes (a swift and unhealthy rise in blood sugar) but also spikes of other nutrients that may be harmful to our bodies. In this case, I'm thinking of calcium, vitamins and fatty acids. Even so, calcification of tissue is one of the leading causes of ageing and death.[12] A sudden influx of calcium and fats may also lead to vascular damage. One potential consequence of these nutrient spikes could be increased concentrations of zinc, copper and iron in the brains of Alzheimer's patients, indicating an unhealthy accumulation of these metals in the body.[13] High doses of magnesium from dietary supplements or medications can also be harmful and can cause nausea, cramps and diarrhoea. Vitamin C spikes could increase the risk of liver damage and vitamin D spikes could contribute to osteoporosis, as vitamin D serves as the signal to the bones to release calcium into the blood. Tryptophan in tablet form can increase the risk of severe muscle pain, nerve damage and skin changes.[14]

All this contradicts the notion of linking healthy eating to chemical terms such as 'saturated fats', 'carbohydrates', 'tryptophan', 'zinc', 'magnesium', 'calcium', 'vitamins', or 'Omega-3 fatty acids', because it is the complexity of whole foods that matters and not individual, isolated nutrients.

Whole foods have a story to tell

Mindful eating enables you to experience the food matrix directly. Right now, as I am writing these lines, I'm biting into a piece of ginger root. The flavour journey begins with warm, woody notes, then moves to bitter, peppery flavours, culminating in that unmistakable ginger kick and a long-lasting, refreshing aftertaste. I rinse my mouth out and then shake a little ground ginger onto my tongue, by way of contrast. It's costly and grown in Cambodia; I bought it from a health food shop in Zurich. With the powder, all the woody, peppery, bitter and refreshing flavours chime in at once, but instead of creating a kind of synergy, there's a general softening of the flavours. I'm experiencing that classic, modern feeling: the boredom of overstimulation.

Cinnamon flowers tell a more thrilling story than ground cinnamon does. Right now, I am slowly chewing three cinnamon flowers and they are taking me on a journey which begins with woody, clove-like flavours, followed by a gentle wave of cinnamon, an interplay of hints of musk, tobacco and thyme, before finishing on a note of refreshing sweetness. By contrast, ground cinnamon offers a two-step flavour experience. First, there is a brief hit of sweetness, then there's that pop of refreshment, like you would have when chewing gum. These two small examples give you an idea of how complex foods with intact food matrices interact with the human organism in a multifaceted way - something that the pop of flavour offered by ground spices or nutrient solutions cannot hope to replicate. That pop of flavour is followed by an emptiness that cries out for further consumption.

Cooking and baking

But if whole foods are so healthy, why do we bother cooking at all? Well, the natural structures of plants and the fibres in animal flesh are so strong that they are challenging – sometimes even impossible – for us to digest. This is tied to the fact that human beings have been grilling, cooking and grinding foods for millennia, performing these transformative processes outside of our bodies to aid our digestion. It is why our guts are relatively small, compared to our brains. When cooking healthy food, for instance, steaming a chicory or sauteing some potatoes, the food's grid-like structures undergo only minimal changes; it becomes a little softer and easier to eat and, as with digestion, new scents, colours and textures emerge. It is thanks to cooking that our brains have grown so large, while our gut and gut flora have remained so small. Cows spend all day chewing and even apes devote six hours to doing the same. Another key element of cooking is that it prevents us from consuming as many harmful bacteria and toxins, which takes the burden off our immune system. It also simply lets us eat much more food – food that we would not be able to digest if it were uncooked. And that's without even mentioning the boost in flavours and the variety of available nutrients unlocked by cooking and baking. Bread, milk chocolate and caramelised carrots are all examples of flavours that are not found in nature; they are human inventions.

The transformation of raw food into cooked food, the gentle transfiguration of the food matrix, is most probably typical of every culture. Cooking has many social benefits. Most animals eat for themselves alone, but cooking brings human beings together, simply because the effort involved naturally invites others to share in the result. Cooking also promotes self-control because we cannot just gobble food down; we must instead consciously choose and prepare what we eat. If you cook, you intuitively avoid adding too much salt, saturated fat and other unhealthy ingredients, which are the order of the day in ready-made and restaurant foods and are used to boost flavour. It's not about pushing ourselves to eat as much as possible and that's why cooking not only makes us more social and more discerning, but also fosters good health.

Keeping and controlling fire were once prerequisites for cooking. One of the most critical insights in human history is our recognition of the fact that cooking requires us to use heat cautiously to preserve the food matrix. We see this in the plethora of words we use to describe heating and processing foods. 'Frying' entails browning the surface of a foodstuff using what is known as the Maillard reaction between proteins and sugars. When the deeper grid-like structures are affected, this is described as 'burning' or 'charring', which is less optimistic. 'Browning' a food involves exposing it to heat for a limited period of time to preserve the internal grid-like structures. 'Sautéing' involves brief exposure to heat and is achieved by tossing the food in a pan. 'Steaming' can be achieved by covering the pot and using a constant, low heat. 'Stewing' uses low heat over a long period to soften foods without breaking down the matrix. When 'poaching' a food, it is essential that both the shape of the food and the food matrix remain intact. 'Flambéing' involves dousing food in alcohol and setting it alight, creating a brief, superficial heat. 'Roasting' and 'grilling' require greater heat over a period of time and are suitable for cooking larger foodstuffs, such as suckling pig, which will retain their anatomical structure despite prolonged exposure to heat.

The amount of heat used has gradually decreased over the history of human cooking culture. Many early humans burned their food to ensure it was free of pathogens. While unhealthy, their consumption of burnt food was balanced by their infrequent cooking and by eating many fruits and other foods raw. Greek mythology bears witness to a great struggle for control of fire. The Greeks were unable to develop cooking until Prometheus stole fire from Zeus after an animal sacrifice. Prometheus's own love of a good intact food matrix is evident from the fact that he ate the juicy and more lightly cooked parts of the sacrificial animal and left the burnt bits to Zeus. His skilful handling of fire made him a pioneer of human civilisation.

At a meal in my student days, I also experienced that ancient sense of pride at having power over fire. A fellow student, an Italian, was cooking spaghetti for us. She was busy talking to us, so she neglected to take the pasta out of the simmering water at the proper moment. Testing it, she decided it wouldn't pass muster. We tried it ourselves and thought it was good, which made her furious. 'It's overcooked!' she cried, throwing the spaghetti in the bin. On the second try, she stood at the stove, constantly glancing at the clock so as not to miss the crucial moment. This time, she was satisfied and the spaghetti was perfectly *al dente*. The mythic pride of Prometheus himself shone in her dark eyes. It taught me what culture and civilisation originally meant, namely, turning raw materials into something healthy. Since the global triumph of processed foods, however, humanity is beginning to let slip the fire and the culture it once so proudly held. And it is doing so not for the benefit of the gods but for industry, which now uses excessive heat to transform complex foods into long-life, amorphous nutrient slime before adding emulsifiers to mould them into pseudofoods. Crisps, margarine and microwave-ready meals have very little in the way of substance.

Industrial pseudofoods are not unhealthy simply because they lack a stable food matrix. Excessive heat from chemical reactions used in cooking can also cause digestive problems.[15] Advanced glycation end products (AGEs), such as those found in mayonnaise, cured meats and hamburger patties, are created through prolonged exposure to dry heat and are particularly problematic. AGEs prompt gut bacteria to produce less butyric acid, which damages the intestinal mucosa and gut bacteria, ultimately leading to digestive disorders. Poor digestion can spawn a vicious cycle: fast food containing AGEs impairs our ability to digest whole foods, which in turn prompts us to consume more fast food containing AGEs. The same vicious cycle can also affect a change in taste preferences. Fast food without a food matrix has a smooth mouth feel; it requires minimal chewing and can be eaten very quickly. To stop this downward spiral, we have to be like Prometheus and regain control of fire by cooking our own pasta and taking responsibility for ensuring that as much of our food as possible is *al dente*.

Noodles are not natural foodstuffs; they are made from semolina or flour, both of which lack a food matrix. Nevertheless, they are believed to contribute to the long lives and good health of people living in the Blue Zones both in the East and in the West. Semolina or flour is mixed with water and kneaded to create a dough, to which other ingredients – such as finely chopped vegetables, eggs or milk – are added. The dough is then rolled out, pressed and shaped. At this point, a small amount of oil is added. Durum wheat, from which Italian pasta is made, contains a lot of gluten. The flour itself feels hard, like sand. Gluten is a wheat protein that forms bonds when exposed to pressure and warmth and creates a matrix that binds other nutrients together – the more of these gluten 'bridges' form, the healthier the dough. Similarly, in breadmaking, gluten is what forms the food matrix. Baking, as a practice, is devoted to building the best gluten-free grids possible. These grids can be observed as large, uniform pores in bread, such as sourdough, which undergoes a lengthy preparation process. Industrial baking, on the other hand, does not take the necessary time to form these gluten grids, meaning that a lot of uncombined gluten remains in the end product, which is a key driver of the increasing rate of gluten intolerance. People who do not have gluten intolerance should not avoid gluten, as bread and pasta produced with emulsifiers to make them gluten-free lack a functioning matrix, which can lead to sugar and insulin spikes and undernourished gut bacteria. You'll notice the absence of a food matrix from the fact that products of this kind are never identifiably *al dente*; they are always soft, even when only briefly heated. In a nutshell, this means that the whole foods rule can be extended to include traditionally produced foods that form a matrix during production. These include *al dente* pasta and traditional breads.

Like whole foods, *al dente* pasta and traditional breads, fermented foods – such as the sauerkraut and yoghurt we encountered in the previous section on the mindful consumption of sour foods – also have a food matrix. In German, fermentation is also called 'kaltgaren' or 'cold cooking', because the process involves live bacteria changing a foodstuff without destroying its matrix. Other health-boosting fermented foods include sourdough bread, gherkins, chocolate, coffee and small amounts of wine and beer. As I mentioned in the section on sour foods, it's best to make fermented foods like yoghurt, kefir, kombucha, sauerkraut, or kimchi yourself, because the products you buy in the supermarket unfortunately tend to contain minimal live cultures.

Canned foods, however, are much better for us than their reputation suggests. Inside a can, the food matrix remains intact, as do healthy nutrients such as polyphenols, which are trapped inside the matrix. Freezing also preserves the matrix of many foodstuffs. There are a few exceptions, of course, such as salad leaves, apples and milk. Sushi chefs advise against freezing raw fish, as it can damage the matrix. Chocolate and truffles are particularly sensitive to cold. On one occasion, I wanted to put some chocolate in the fridge and my grandfather nearly went berserk.

In light of this, the discovery of the crucial importance of the food matrix to nutritional medicine, ought to have radical consequences for pharmacies and drug stores. If it is simply a matter of eating healthily, these shops should stop selling nutrient powders and instead sell whole plants. You'd soon be unable to tell them apart from your average fruit or vegetable market. Pharmacists selling whole foods would remind their customers that on no account should they put them through the blender and any packaging would read: 'Simply wash before eating. Do not peel. Enjoy slowly and mindfully.'

The importance of nutritional diversity

As I have said, there is a tendency to view healthy eating as a simple combination of macro and micronutrients.

One problem with this definition of healthy eating is the lack of consideration afforded to the food matrix. The second problem is the failure to consider nutritional diversity. At present, food labels suggest that all carbohydrates, all proteins and all fats are equal, which is clearly untrue. Margarine containing trans fats is not on a par with cold-pressed olive oil from Italy, Greece, or Spain. Our bodies respond to the two in completely different ways. Protein from a piece of wild salmon is not the same as protein from highly processed mince. Carbohydrates in sugar are not the same as carbohydrates from onions and celery.

Not all calories were created equal. The calories in sugar cause insulin spikes and the formation of fat deposits, whereas calories from fat and whole foods are less likely to do so. Calories, which are integrated in a food matrix, are less likely to make a person gain weight than calories in a nutrient solution; the calories in salads are less likely to prompt weight gain than the calories in biscuits. Indeed, we often do not know the precise composition and number of calories in whole foods, but this is not a problem. We can learn how likely they are to provoke weight gain without knowing the exact chemical mechanisms. And they are always the healthier choice. However, since we are not always able to choose whole foods, it's helpful to know that the total calorie count and sugar content are the most important pieces of information on any food label.

The industry's wishful thinking

When it comes to micronutrients, the industry suggests that we concentrate on the essentials, which it, unlike our bodies, can produce in large quantities. Yet we are not suffering from a lack of essential nutrients; these are abundant in whole foods (and fast food). The fertilisers used in agriculture contain increasingly high levels of micronutrients such as magnesium, zinc and copper, leading to higher levels of these in our food. Similarly, many foods and drinks are fortified with these essential nutrients, such that, taken together, all this can easily lead to high intakes of certain micronutrients, the potential consequences of which could include hypervitaminosis, vascular calcification and dementia. An example of this is Omega-3 fatty acids, which are found in fish and are considered essential because our bodies cannot produce them independently. About ten years ago, I took a particular interest in the research into Omega-3 fatty acids and used them to treat patients suffering from depression. However, after looking more closely into these fatty acids, I have stopped recommending them as a treatment.

Even the manufacturers' adverts, which claim that many people are suffering from a lack of Omega-3 fatty acids, may not be true for all individuals. Our metabolism can make Omega-3 fatty acids not just from animal fats but also from plant fats. A single tablespoon of rapeseed oil contains enough alpha-linolenic acid to ensure our body can meet its daily needs for Omega-3 fatty acids. In addition, many studies have shown the potential harm of taking Omega-3 fatty acids as nutritional supplements and actively advise against it. One of the most extensive studies to date on the health effects of Omega-3 fatty acids, the DART-II study, found that consuming the fatty acids as a nutritional supplement is not only unnecessary but could be potentially harmful, raising the risk of early cardiac death by 27 per cent.[16] Taking Omega-3 fatty acids in pregnancy also led to an increased incidence of behavioural problems in children.[17] Another study of over 18,000 Americans demonstrated that Omega-3 fatty acids do not improve depressive symptoms but exacerbate them.[18] Then there are the ecological problems caused by the manufacture of these supplements. Yet treatments involving fish oil capsules have now become an industry in themselves, pulling in more than thirty-three billion US dollars annually. More than an eighth of the fish caught worldwide are used to produce nutritional supplements, which are neither pleasurable to consume nor do anything to promote good health.[20]

Here are three examples of misinformation which benefit the chemicals industry by helping them to extol the supposed health benefits of their artificial supplements:

- **What the industry's wishful thinking would have you think:** fish is healthy because it contains Omega-3 fatty acids.
- **What the science says:** fish is healthy due to the thousands of nutrients it contains, integrated

within a food matrix. We still have not identified many of these nutrients and cannot manufacture them on an industrial scale.

• **What the industry's wishful thinking would have you think:**sunlight is healthy because it provides us with vitamin D.

• **What the science says:** Vitamin D is ineffective where there is minimal sunlight and harmful in very high doses. Sunlight is healthy due to its many effects, some of which we still do not understand, including setting our internal clock and regulating the serotonin and melatonin systems that are responsible for our biological rhythms.

• **What the industry's wishful thinking would have you think:** whole fruits are healthy because they contain vitamin C.

• **What the science says:** studies have shown vitamin C to be ineffective when it comes to cancer, heart conditions and ageing. Whole fruits are healthy because they contain thousands of antioxidants – many of which we still have not identified – and the nutrients and fibre they contain exhibit a three-dimensional structure that promotes mindful eating and slow and steady digestion.

Alternatives to industrial nutrient supplements

But what are the alternatives to the industry's wishful thinking, which likes to pass itself off as science? One example is Hildegard von Bingen's concept of the greening power, a concept of health that emphasises the importance of diversity. Hildegard conceived of the greening power as a substance present in the soil which, given moisture and warmth, rises into the leaves of plants via the roots. It is why she sometimes also referred to the greening power as the root-force. In her recipes, she recommended combining different fresh, green and readily available herbs, roughly chopping them and mixing them with flour, olive oil, water, wine, vinegar and honey and seasoning them with ginger, nutmeg, pepper and cinnamon. She considered garden plants such as dill, fennel, fenugreek, sage, poppy, oregano, aloe, rue, verbena, cinquefoil, parsley, wormwood and basil to be particularly healthy and she would also forage for centaury, stinging nettles, bay, mint, mallow and wild geranium.

On his travels in Italy, Goethe was inspired by the variety and quantity of vegetables used in Italian cuisine. In May 1787, he wrote in his diary: '[…] indeed, the Neapolitans consume so many vegetables that the leaves of cauliflowers, broccoli, artichokes, cabbages, lettuce and garlic make up the greater part of the city's refuse. Two large, flexible panniers are slung over the back of a donkey: these are not only filled to the brim, but above them towers a huge mound of refuse, piled with peculiar cunning. No garden could exist without a donkey.'[20] I experienced the sheer variety of Asian food for myself on my travels through China and Taiwan. Every starter, every soup and every side dish I enjoyed was a balance of sweet, sour, salty, bitter and savoury flavours, the entire cosmos of Chinese cooking in a single bite. When I visited the National Palace Museum in Taipei, home to 620,000 precious objects of incalculable worth, I was led to the museum's most treasured piece. It was housed in a cabinet made of thick glass and surrounded by numerous other visitors, so catching a glimpse of the piece required some patience. It was a green cabbage, carved from a single piece of jadeite. Its leaves looked distinctly realistic, each with a slightly different shape, colour gradient and texture. Natural brown marks highlighted the sculptor's attention to detail. It was a veritable celebration of the food matrix and its diversity. The museum's second-most popular piece was on show across from the cabbage: a piece of jasper that so resembled a piece of Dongpo braised pork belly that you had to look very close to be sure that it was in fact stone and not meat. Dongpo pork belly is an umami-rich delicacy in China. It is made using a tender piece of pork belly, slow-cooked in a blend of fresh ginger, fragrant spring onions, savoury soya sauce and aromatic rice wine. The traditional recipe can be traced back to the great Chinese poet, painter and politician, Su Shi (1037–1101), whose satirical poems about the government led to him being banished to Hubei province, where he gained his pen name Dongpo (after a farm where he spent a lot of time). Instead of growing melancholy and bitter, he found happiness in the kitchen and in the pursuit of food that was truly nourishing. During his years in exile, he created several dishes, from Dongpo pork belly to a spiced cucumber salad. Both dishes place great emphasis on the richness of flavour and culinary diversity.

It's an approach shared by the five elements of

Chinese cuisine, which are rooted in the principles of traditional Chinese medicine. Each food is assigned to one of the five elements (earth, wood, fire, metal and water), each of which is believed to have a particular effect on the flows of energy in the body. These rankings are based on the temperature and flavour intensity of each food (sweet, sour, bitter, spicy and salty). In contrast to the industrialised theories in the West, which reduce food to mere nutrients, the Chinese concept promotes conscious, mindful eating. The aim is to take a long-term route through the five elements, maintaining the body's balance of energies by consuming the greatest possible variety of nutrients and flavours. For instance, one meal might include beetroot as the sweet earth element, lemon as the sour wood element, salad as the bitter fire element, onions as the spicy metal element and prawns as the salty water element. Fresh, seasonal ingredients are preferred because they are believed to act in greater harmony with the body. The nutritional concept of 'eating the rainbow', which encourages people to consume a variety of colourful fruits and vegetables, is related to this kind of cuisine. Each colour represents a group of nutrients that offer holistic benefits to the body, such as lycopene-like substances in red tomatoes, minerals in green spinach and antioxidants in purple berries.

In the past decade, nutritional diversity has become an established concept in medical research, due in part to the discovery that a variety of gut flora can protect against ailments such as obesity, diabetes, autoimmune diseases, depression, bowel cancer and dementia. And the variety of bacteria present depends significantly on the diversity of the food consumed. It does not appear to matter for the diversity of the microbiome whether you are an omnivore or a vegetarian. What matters is the number of different plant species that you eat. Participants in a study who ate more than 30 plant species per week had particularly diverse gut bacteria.[21] Eating muesli for breakfast, with a mix of oats, raisins, apples, pears, bananas, raspberries, blueberries, strawberries, hazelnuts and walnuts, gives you ten plant species straight out of the gate. A lunch of vegetable stew containing onions, celery, tomatoes, beans, aubergines, potatoes, carrots, broccoli, cauliflower and pumpkin seeds gets you to twenty. Then, for dinner, you might have a salad made of three varieties of leaves: lettuce, dandelion and chicory, plus sweetcorn, olives, cucumber, pine nuts, sunflower seeds and orange segments and that brings you to thirty in a single day. And if you want to give your gut bacteria an extra boost, you can reach for fermented foods like sauerkraut, kefir, kombucha, yoghurt, or kimchi, which also help to prevent unnecessary inflammatory responses in the gut.[22]

The dwindling variety of plant species we consume is becoming a problem.

The dramatic drop in the number of species that we eat is problematic and may also be another significant driver of the increase in many diseases. For example, there are 7,500 varieties of apples in nature, but the selection at the supermarket is far narrower. Every apple has twice as many genes as a human. These genes give apples a wide range of chemical compounds that are essential for energy, a fresh appearance and protection against pests. The diversity of their genes also explains the many different rates at which different apples ripen and the vast diversity of taste and texture. Every variety also contains various quantities of polyphenols and nutrients, so it is worth keeping an eye out for rare and unusual fruits and vegetables at markets and specialist shops.

'Even the honey I produce myself has lost its colour and tastes increasingly dull and my swarms of bees are losing their vitality!' a friend of mine complained one day. He had been keeping bees and producing honey for decades. The diversity of our soils, meadows and forests is dropping, which means that our food is becoming less diverse, too. It might contain higher levels of nitrogen, magnesium, copper and phosphorus. Yet it lacks thousands of other nutrients that we cannot easily manufacture or add to our diets or to the fertilisers we use. This drop in diversity is easy to see and taste in honey.

Honey is composed of over 200 key components and over 500 volatile compounds, which only reveal themselves when the honey is eaten, lending it its unique taste and scent. Its matrix is relatively weak, which is why it is best consumed in small quantities. The many and varied nutrients it contains are potentially crucial for our health, including polyphenols, organic acids, aromatic compounds and enzymes. The variety of these nutrients depends on what the bees eat. If the flora in the area the bees inhabit is monotonous, this will be reflected in the honey, which will contain a narrower range of nutrients. In my friend's case, the use of fertilisers in his local area led to the disappearance of diverse, colourful grassland.

The loss of colour in his bees' honeycombs can be traced back to a reduction in the diversity of nearby pollens. Even so, my friend's honey is still worlds away from the cheap honey you get at the supermarket. Incidentally, a third of the honey sold in the EU is an imitation, composed almost entirely of sugar, so it makes sense to buy it straight from the beekeeper.

Food is an important source of inspiration, so when our food is impoverished, we become culturally and spiritually impoverished, too. The wild honey that John the Baptist tasted in the desert marked the beginning of his radical transformation; he turned towards spiritual nourishment, which truly nourished him and brought him enlightenment. In the Indian Upanisads, the wise teacher Uddālaka Āruṇi introduced his son Śvetaketu Auddālaki to the spiritual secret of the unity of all being by showing him a swarm of bees:

'Now, take the bees, son. They prepare the honey by gathering nectar from a variety of trees and reducing it to a homogeneous whole. In that state, the nectar from each different tree is not able to differentiate: 'I am the nectar of that tree' and 'I am the nectar of this tree.'[23] The mystical unity of humanity and the cosmos is made manifest to Śvetaketu through the unified diversity of honey. A sugar water solution, enriched with a bit of zinc, selenium and artificial flavours, cannot offer the same kind of experience; it leaves only emptiness behind.

Medicinal plants: hope for holistic medicine?

In light of the above, I am very pleased to see that new, scientifically superior studies have at least confirmed the efficacy of medicinal plants. These plants do not work like medicines, via a single chemical substance, but use a variety of substances which take shape within the plant matrix. Ginkgo remedies are made from the leaves of the ginkgo tree, which can live for over a thousand years. The hundreds of active ingredients that ginkgo contains include ginkgolides, flavone glycosides and terpenoids, which promote blood flow in the brain, inhibit blood clotting and have antioxidant properties. Circulatory disorders and oxidative stress contribute significantly towards brain ageing, so this plant remedy has the potential to protect the brain, improve memory and prevent dementia. However, ginkgo biloba should only be taken under medical supervision due to possible side effects such as seizures, haemorrhage and interactions with other medications.

Lavender oil is another plant remedy that Hildegard von Bingen used to treat ailments. A few years ago, it was officially approved as a treatment for restlessness and anxious mood. Again, the effects of lavender oil cannot be traced back to individual ingredients, such as linalool and linalyl acetate. Instead, it is the ingredients as a whole which appear to account for its beneficial effects. It's also a stroke of luck that lavender oil isn't addictive, as other sedatives are. Diversity knows no dependency.

The antidepressant effects of St John's wort (which is banned in some countries and available only by prescription in others), a popular remedy since antiquity, have now been confirmed in a series of clinical studies. We do not know precisely which of its ingredients are responsible for its curative effects. It is assumed that at least seven individual substances are at work, if not more. Its modulatory effects on various messenger systems, including those for serotonin, dopamine, noradrenaline, GABA and glutamate, are similarly varied. Tolerance of St John's wort is generally better than that of conventional antidepressants; however, it can cause sensitivity to light and should not be taken alongside other medicines, particularly HIV medication and immunomodulators.

Alongside the success of herbal remedies, research into live bacteria has also yielded promising findings. Medications containing a variety of bacteria appear to support good health. One recently published study showed that bacteria can reduce depression symptoms, using a probiotic comprising fourteen different strains of bacteria: four different bifidobacteria, eight different species of lactobacillus, one strain of streptococcus and one of bacillus subtilis.[24]

While there is increasing evidence supporting the importance of variety in natural remedies, as with food, there is still insufficient research on whether the matrix of plant remedies plays a significant role in their therapeutic effects. Studies show that herbal remedies, which lack a matrix and are administered as extracts and oils, can exert an effect solely due to their diversity. However, I would not rule out the possibility that a matrix could have additional effects, because it encourages more intensive digestion, intensifying the interactions between any given remedy and our bodies.

It's why I like to open plant remedy capsules to get a closer look. Larger leaves or plant pieces suggest a higher-quality product. And I would not be at all surprised if the probiotics in foods such as sauerkraut and yoghurt proved more effective than those in sachets or tablets.

In this chapter, I have aimed to present a new theory of nutrition that aligns with recent scientific findings. It explains the health-harming potential of essential nutrient solutions and the dangers posed by highly processed foods and accounts for why colourful blends of solid and whole foods come off best in studies investigating how best to promote good health.

The following points seem to me to be of most significant importance:

- Our bodies have millions of years of experience with whole foods, which has led to a multi-stage digestive process in which the food matrix is broken down step by step and new nutrients emerge.
- Consequently, not all calories are created equal.

Calories from processed foods may lead to increased weight gain because they are not integrated into a matrix and behave as 'naked' calories, triggering a significant insulin response.

• Carbohydrates are not all created equal, either. Even people with diabetes can eat fruit, because the complex plant matrix incorporates the fruit's simple sugars in such a way that the body is better able to tolerate them. Even potatoes are better than their reputation would have you believe, because their sugars take the form of long chains contained within a matrix.

• Nor are fats created equal. Fats can also form a matrix which incorporates sugars. However, low-fat processed foods often contain added sugar to make them more palatable. This is particularly harmful because this sugar then enters the bloodstream unchecked.

• Plant proteins are not at a disadvantage when compared to animal proteins, as long as we observe the fundamental principle of diversity and eat a combination of grains, seeds, nuts and beans.

• Fermented foods are particularly healthy if they exhibit a crunchy matrix and contain a variety of probiotics.

• Dried, frozen or tinned whole foods can still be healthy, providing their matrix is intact and they do not contain chemical additives and large quantities of salt or sugar.

• The loss of sense of smell sometimes observed in old age is not a natural process but is instead the result of unbalanced and industrially processed food, which also accelerates ageing.[25] Mindful eating is the most effective way of breaking this vicious cycle.

•	Modern science has confirmed the therapeutic value of plant remedies, such as St John's wort and lavender oil, the effects of which are due to the abundance of medicinal substances they contain.

EATING RITUALS AND EATING IN COMPANY

In the previous chapter, we learned about how important it is to consider the food matrix and the diversity of foods more generally when cooking. In this chapter, we will look more closely at the practice of eating in company, in which food takes a central role in relationships, culture and spirituality.

As a teenager, Esther – a patient of mine – suffered from terrible stomach aches after every meal. A series of investigations at a university hospital revealed that her stomach and small intestine were not moving. She has had to be fed intravenously ever since, and, as I mentioned in the previous chapter, this comes with numerous medical disadvantages. Unlike Claudia, whose story I shared in the introduction and who quickly deteriorated and died while being fed intravenously, Esther has tolerated this form of feeding much better. She is happy to no longer suffer from her previous stomach aches. Yet even in her case, the treatment is not without its issues. She has complained not just of physical ailments such as exhaustion and weakness, but social ones too: 'I'm excluded from social life. When you don't eat, you don't have friends. Or a boyfriend. No one wants to be friends with me, because I can't eat.' Put yourself in Esther's shoes for a moment: no birthday cakes, no Christmas dinner, no romantic dinner dates.

Esther's story reveals that food is much more than just the consumption of nutrients, particularly when we eat together. It is a process that sees food move from a position outside the body to one inside, yet, at the same time, this process of internalisation and integration takes place on an interpersonal level. There is probably no way of forming a group that is more effective than eating together. It's no coincidence that food and drink are important symbols and markers of identity in every culture. The way that food and drink are shared between people often indicates the strength of the bond between them. Drinks without a meal are noncommittal and well-suited to fostering interactions between strangers or mere acquaintances. By contrast, a meal with drinks is reserved for close acquaintances, friends and special guests. Similarly, family cohesion is strengthened through shared meals. Wedding celebrations and birthday parties centre on an elaborately decorated cake and decadent dinners and sweet treats are key features of Christmas celebrations. On the Trobriand Islands of Papua New Guinea, sex before marriage is permitted, but eating together is not. This rule is a striking example of how important it is to eat together for family cohesion. But it's not just in older cultures and family traditions where eating together plays a central role; it is also experiencing a renaissance in reality TV shows like *Survivor* and *Big Brother*. In these situations, as in ancient eating rituals, it fosters social cohesion, serves as a stage for conflict and drama and contributes significantly to the programme's emotional depth.

Communal meals are also a good opportunity to understand a key aspect of spirituality. Consider the following paradox: in Aboriginal cultures, at a traditional meal with hosts and guests, the number of calories available per person decreases as more people sit down at the table. Without community spirit, which often has a spiritual element, this would be considered a significant disadvantage. The more people at the table, the worse off they all are. In reality, however, we see the exact opposite: eating together is more joyful than eating alone, and the effect of communal eating is so profound that many people struggle emotionally with solo eating, even though it means that all the calories before them are up for grabs. The questionable enjoyment of having sole control over all the calories on offer is evident in the fact that television, smartphones and newspapers often accompany solo eating. The joy of sharing calories seems, therefore, to be greater than the pleasure of consuming calories. The multiplication of food that we see time and again in the Bible alludes to this notion of shared joy. Indeed, there is an anticapitalist element to eating together: it's not about grabbing the most significant portion as quickly as you can to increase your own calorific capital. A good dining companion is patient, happy to share, sets their differences aside before the meal, waits for the others to start and stays at the table until everyone has finished. Eating together counteracts the contradiction that capitalism undermines and destroys the trust, courtesy and good manners on which it depends.

Alongside its social and spiritual advantages, eating together also benefits our health. In the first chapter, I described how mindful eating can activate the vagus nerve. The latest studies have shown that this effect is even more pronounced when we eat mindfully *together*.[1] Interestingly enough, this is reflected in the concept of the diet, which is much more multifaceted than is generally assumed. The ancient Greek 'diaita' means 'lifestyle' or 'way of living'.

The term 'diet' is also related to the much older word 'diaitáo', meaning an intensive giving, taking and sharing. Other ancient Greek words related to 'diet', such as 'dais' and 'daínu', refer to both eating and sharing. This proves that the original concept of a diet encompassed far more than a selection of suitable nutrients. It was much more about sharing and the social ties that food might impart.[2] It's no coincidence, then, that people in the Blue Zones, like Sister André and Kane Tanaka, not only eat mindfully and healthily, but also eat in the company of others.

Communal eating and psychological issues

The significant social element that eating entails can also be observed in eating disorders, which, unfortunately, often contribute to interpersonal issues and isolation. Bulimia is characterised by episodes of binge eating and unhealthy methods of weight reduction, such as vomiting, laxatives, or excessive sport. Those suffering from the condition can experience such severe hunger that they prefer not to share food, to have all the available calories to themselves. This greed and the feelings of shame associated with it cause the person to withdraw socially and hide the eating disorder. In cases of anorexia, the sufferer's pride at being able to forego calories prevents them from integrating into communal eating situations. The unifying power of a shared appetite is alien to them. If they force themselves to eat, gastrointestinal issues and feelings of shame and guilt will likely stifle any potential enjoyment. By the same token, social problems such as rejection, bullying and emotional and sexual abuse can be key causes of eating disorders and obesity. Not only is this connection proven by studies, but it is also hinted at by several idioms: 'I had to chew it over', 'They left me to stew', 'He buttered me up'.

Max was a young man with a passion for numbers and an extraordinary musical talent. I got to know him as part of an investigation into his eating habits. His love of numbers, along with his perceptiveness and sensitivity, brought him happiness from time to time, but it also brought challenges, particularly in social situations and around eating. Even in his early years, Max showed signs of sensitivity to certain textures and flavours. Eating was often unpleasant for him, which led him to avoid many foods and left him feeling uncomfortable at the dinner table. Because he had been diagnosed with autism, his parents were very understanding and tried to fulfil his every wish. The consequence of this, however, was that he only ever ate alone and at irregular times, typically eating squares of processed cheese, soft white bread and chocolate. His disordered eating habits contributed to his sense of social isolation because he felt ashamed of them.

Despite his diagnosis of autism, Max had highly advanced social skills. He was visibly happy in our sessions. He deliberately directed my attention to the pictures of human faces on my desk – a behaviour rather untypical of autism. I cast doubt on his diagnosis and recommended that Max's parents eat with him and work to diversify his diet gradually. This was an enormous change for his parents; they had grown used to seeing Max as in need of help and accommodating him at every turn. I helped them to be more active and resolute in their parenting and establish a structured menu. What was interesting was that Max wasn't upset with me, even though his new diet gave him stomach issues and diarrhoea at first and adapting to eating healthy food, including whole fruits and vegetables, was a slow process that took a lot of getting used to. He told me, 'You sussed me out somehow and it's not a nice feeling, but it had to happen sometime.' In therapy, not only did his eating habits eventually improve, but his social life did too. He joined a table tennis club and was prepared to meet up with the people he met there for food and drinks, rather than interact with them online.

As Max's story illustrates, eating together plays a central role in treating social isolation and eating disorders. Yet therapy does not always go this smoothly. If parents can't participate, be it for want of time or due to their own eating disorders and the family does not have a habit of eating together, therapy becomes more laborious. In cases such as these, specialised eating disorder clinics can be an invaluable option, offering an element of peer pressure and professional support, even in cases of severely disordered eating. Sometimes, however, a retreat will do the job, establishing the social pressure to eat regularly and in company. However, prevention is always easier and more effective than a cure. Eating together with children lowers the risk of mental and physical lifestyle diseases. Family rituals are essential for mindful eating and for maintaining a pattern of eating later in life. The more secure a child's social bonds are, the easier it will be for them to accept – or indeed refuse – food from other people.[3]

Historians generally assume that cooking and eating together marked the beginning of human culture. Presumably, the first human words referred to eating, just like the ancient word 'diet'. When we eat, we experience our own frailties, our secret desire, our appetite, all of which unite us. Expressions like 'eating humble pie', 'to cut the mustard' and 'knowing which side your bread is buttered' are proof of how deeply connected food and social life have been and continue to be. To a certain extent, eating together is the precursor to psychotherapy. He might have done so a little late, but Max was ultimately able to experience this, the origin of all culture, together with his parents.

Communal eating and the love hormone

Sharing food is not only an outstanding cultural achievement, but it also presents a hormonal challenge and an opportunity. Animals eat alone or in groups, but only human beings truly dine together. Animals experience a physiological trade-off between eating and social behaviour. Hunger neurons suppress social interests, making the animal more concerned with eating. The release of hormones such as leptin and neurotensin encourages movement, social contact and sexuality by suppressing hunger.[4] This interplay is particularly marked in owls. Male owls demonstrate their readiness to mate by offering the females food, which requires them to tolerate their own hunger. This show of generosity is rewarded with sex. The ability to suppress hunger is also a sign that the owl is ready to take on the role of father and provide food for the family.

In human eroticism, however, hunger does not play a decisive role. Instead, it is shared appetites, the experience of culinary pleasures together and the sharing of culinary skills that stimulate hormones such as oxytocin, leptin and neurotensin, fostering a deeper connection and attraction. The German fairytale *The Man without a Heart* impressively illustrates this. An older man has been living without a heart. He confesses to his young housekeeper that his heart is inside a bird which is refusing food and is trapped in an ancient church. Desperate to help the older man find love, the housekeeper tells his secret to an attractive young wanderer who decides to search for the bird. The housekeeper packs him plenty of food and drink and wishes him luck. On his journey, he sits on the ground to eat his meals and calls out, 'Well, well, time for a feast! Come join and be my guest!' His first guest is an ox who tucks in and says, 'A great many thanks to you and should you need someone to help when you're in need or in danger, simply call out to me, your guest.' His second guest is a pig, which takes its leave, saying: 'Many thanks and when your life is on the line, be sure to call for this swine!' His third guest is a great bird, which eats and says, 'If you need me, just call for me!' All three of the wanderer's guests keep their word. The great bird leads the wanderer to the church, where the trapped bird is fluttering around in desperation. However, a deep moat surrounds the church and the wanderer cannot cross it. Yet the grateful ox hurries to the wanderer's aid and drinks the moat dry in a single gulp. The final hurdle is the thick church wall, which has no doors or windows. This is where the pig comes eagerly running in and uses its tusks to dig a hole under the church wall. The wanderer slips through, catches the starving bird and gives it to the housekeeper. Just as he is finishing the last bite of the provisions he took on his journey, sharing them with the housekeeper, the bird finds its appetite and tucks in. In that moment, the older man is redeemed and closes his eyes for the last time. The young woman falls in love with the generous wanderer, who was so happy to share his feast and they live happily ever after.

The Oscar-winning film *Babette's Feast*, based on a story by Karen Blixen, illustrates the unifying power of communal dining. The story unfolds in the nineteenth century in a far-flung Danish coastal town, where the devout local congregation is presided over by the daughters of the late pastor. The congregation avoids indulgence and limits itself to simple, bland food. Despite the group's deep Christian convictions, tensions, jealousy and resentments come to the fore. One day, a woman named Babette arrives, having fled France and asks the sisters for work and lodging. In time, she gains the sisters' trust and they come to value her commitment and support. When Babette wins 10,000 francs in a French lottery, she decides to use the money to host an opulent feast that ultimately transforms the congregation. It is fascinating to watch Babette build bridges and restore lost connections through food, despite her outsider status. By lovingly preparing a feast, she opens the congregation's hearts and helps them to overcome their differences. The film poignantly underlines the transformative and unifying effects of food prepared with passion and love on both social and spiritual levels.

The psychology of eating together

The hormones that are stimulated when we eat together have an impact on the psyche. Robin Dunbar, a British psychologist at Oxford University, conducted a fascinating study of the practice of eating together.[5] He was able to prove that eating together helps people to build trust in one another – a typical effect of oxytocin. This leads to greater personal interactions and facilitates the development of interpersonal relationships. According to the study, this effect does not depend on people specifically, but on mealtimes.

People tend to feel particularly close to the people they eat dinner with, because it is the daily meal that is least likely to be time-restricted, lacks an outward goal and often involves greater alcohol consumption, which also fosters social interaction (more on this at the end of the chapter). If you want to build a closer rapport with people, the best approach is to invite them to dinner.

Dunbar also discovered that the more people are present at a meal, the more likely they are to laugh and indulge in nostalgia. So, if you gather a small group for dinner and the mood is off, it may be wise to invite more people, especially those who are naturally upbeat.

It can also be a good idea for bosses and managers deemed too detached or narcissistic to eat with their colleagues. People who eat together tend to find each other more pleasant and more sympathetic than they would otherwise and to view each other as equals. Dominant and submissive behaviours tend to decrease at the dinner table, in favour of amenable behaviours. On the other hand, if you, as a boss, have trouble commanding respect and asserting yourself, it may help to avoid eating with colleagues and instead meet with them one-to-one for conversations with clear goals.

Eating together is also a good opportunity to gain a deeper understanding of those you don't understand, or can't quite work out, or by whom you yourself do not feel well understood, because eating together involves intense physical experiences and actions and it is harder to hide than it would be during an everyday conversation. Mirror neurons are an essential part of our capacity for physical perception and they become active both when we act and when we observe others performing a similar action. Eating together is a veritable fiesta for mirror neurons; the surfeit of similar movements of arms, hands and face muscles sends them into a frenzy. It's a good thing, too, because these neurons help us get to know and understand the person across from us on a physical and intuitive level. This is evident in the fact that conversations and interactions in these settings tend to be more direct, lively and personal. In the long term, this means that the person with whom we interact through mirror neurons appears less alien to us and becomes easier to understand. It also explains why Claudia and Esther, whose gastrointestinal issues made it impossible for them to eat with other people, felt excluded not just from the pleasures of food but from life more generally. In turn, this sense of loneliness negatively impacted their health.

Scent: a social glue?

Scent plays a vital role in social cohesion. At the dinner table, the scents of individual dishes blend with the scents of those sitting down to eat. Over time, this causes food preferences to converge and gut bacteria to harmonise. It explains why sitting down to eat together can provide lifelong stability and contribute to a sense of cultural identity. The precursor to the practice of eating together is pregnancy, during which a mother can permanently shape her child simply with her own scents and food preferences. This has been the subject of much research, particularly in the case of a fondness for garlic, which is passed on to the child via its mother's milk.

However, the time a child spends at its mother's breast is not only necessary for passing on a love of all things garlicky; it is also crucial for generating a sense of belonging and trust in food and people. Newborns have a perfect sense of smell, which enables them to recognise trusted people. At just six weeks of age, babies can already distinguish between the taste of their mother's breasts and other breasts. Mothers also find their own children's scent pleasant and prefer it to that of other children. The connection between the attractive scents of other people and the smells of various foods is clear when we consider that many popular perfumes smell like foodstuffs. They often contain vanilla, lemon, orange, bergamot, mandarin, grapefruit, coconut, almond, extracts from green tea, black tea, chamomile, mint and cucumber. The Bible says that the Persian king Ahasuerus' concubines would spend twelve months perfuming themselves with the most delicious scents before receiving him.

But it's not just children; the scents we experience when eating together have a unifying effect on adults. Scents are an important anchor for memory and help us to remember the times we shared with our dining companions in the long term. Meals with intense smells, such as a roast, are more likely to foster memories than less fragrant foods, such as water and ice cream. It's no coincidence that good-smelling bread is Christianity's preferred method for binding people together. Acquaintances of mine who know a thing or two about selling property go so far as to recommend baking a loaf of bread before prospective buyers arrive; the smell of freshly baked bread increases the likelihood that they will feel at home and makes them all the readier to pay a reasonable price.

People who are less adept at picking up scents are shut out of these subtle interactions. People who suffered from olfactory disorders following infection with COVID-19 were shown to eat more fast food and lose their previous eating patterns. Their social relationships also suffered; they exhibited less empathy and were increasingly perceived as distant and impersonal, which contributed to a sense of frustration, anxiety, depression and social isolation. People who are born with a poor sense of smell also suffer from these problems. Overall, they tend to have fewer friends, are less close to family members and spend more time alone.[6] However, people who exhibit a perfect sense of smell and find the slightest hint of perfume or bad breath unpleasantly intense and overwhelming also suffer from social withdrawal and poor diet, because, for them, smells do not foster a sense of belonging but instead provoke disgust and cause stress.

All these findings show that smell plays a vital role in how we feel comfortable and at home. Not only is this connection deeply rooted in our personal lives, but it is also embedded in the story of evolution itself.

Salmon are a striking example of this. They begin their lives in rivers and spend most of their adult lives in the sea before returning, at the end of their lives, to their place of birth to spawn. As young fish, they form a kind of scent memory which helps them to find their way back later in life. It is also assumed that elephants undertake long treks to the habitats where they spent their childhood, because they possess chemical memories of vegetation, minerals, watering holes and even the scent of the rain.

The role of gut bacteria in facilitating relationships

The bacteria in our gut also play an essential role in forming scent communities. The longer and more closely we live and eat with others, the more similar our gut bacteria become. The same is true for our food preferences and the smell of our bodies.[7] The larger and more diverse the group of people we sit down to eat with, the more varied our gut bacteria become, which, in turn, boosts the sense of joy we take from social situations and bolsters our openness to social interaction.

Studies on identical twins demonstrate that digestion and body weight depend more on the gut bacteria we exchange with one another than on genes. This means that the people we sit down to eat with are a key influence on our long-term appetite and metabolism.[8] These new scientific findings have kindled hopes that numerous conditions, including obesity, depression, autism and autoimmune diseases, could be improved by an exchange of gut bacteria.

The following examples demonstrate just how great the need to connect with other people and animals via gut bacteria has become. Kathy High, an American artist with Crohn's disease, an inflammatory bowel condition, decided to try a faecal transplant treatment, a medical intervention which involves the stool of a healthy donor being transplanted into the patient's gut, to enrich their microbiome. This method has already seen success in cases of some gastrointestinal infections. The difficulty is finding a healthy donor. Who exactly is truly healthy? Who is guaranteed not to be carrying disease-fostering bacteria in their gut? High decided to go looking for the stool herself and went so far as to ask a man she deeply admired: David Bowie. She sent him a few photos of herself dressed as him to prove how much of a fan she was. Unfortunately, Bowie died before he was able to reply. The Canadian artist and biologist, François-Joseph Lapointe, had a similarly unusual fixation: he travelled to Guinea to collect bat droppings, his favourite animals and had them transplanted into his gut. He claimed that this method enabled him to think up and perform a 'bat dance'. Both examples demonstrate just how much new findings on gut bacteria have stimulated the imagination, even if the experiments themselves were rather unserious and ought on no account to be repeated at home.

After extensive investigation, a friend of mine also underwent a gut bacteria treatment. A successful biochemist and university professor, he had suffered from gastrointestinal infections since childhood and had several allergies, including to eggs and flower pollen. After undergoing a faecal transplant at the Taymount Clinic in the UK, he experienced a significant and sustained improvement in his symptoms. He can now eat eggs again and has not had any infections since the treatment. This is a single case and is certainly not a study of any kind, but it is still a helpful example. He told me he was convinced that anaerobic bacteria were key to his health problems. Anaerobic bacteria cannot be cultivated in a laboratory and are not present in any probiotics because they cannot tolerate oxygen. The reason this method of transplanting bacteria is not widespread is, in part, due to the difficulty of finding suitable donors and their potential for severe side effects. Until these issues are resolved, it is best to rely on natural methods of bacterial exchange, with eating together being key among these. Incidentally, Swiss fondue is particularly effective for this because everyone eats from the same pot. The people who sit down together to eat enrich the probiotics in the cheese with their own diverse set of bacteria.

Flavour communities

When it comes to eating together, flavour and chemistry are as key as smell and hormonal and psychological factors. If everyone is drinking wine while I sip chamomile tea, I feel left out. And if everyone is enjoying a roast with potatoes and I've just got a pile of raw vegetables on my plate, my sense of unity with the people I am dining with is limited. When it comes to alcohol, there's a simple explanation. Alcohol enhances the effects of the calming brain chemical gamma-aminobutyric acid, or GABA, which prompts the brain to slow down and become disinhibited, as well as leading to more emotional thinking. All this is highly conducive to a sense of cosiness and conviviality. If you do find yourself in similarly booze-tinged company and you're only drinking a chamomile tea, you will often struggle to feel in sync with those around you and interact on the same mental level. A similar situation will occur with caffeine, which awakens and speeds up the brain. It's why herbal tea drinkers might feel like listless outsiders in the company of coffee drinkers.

The extent to which similar foods determine social coordination is less well researched because we still know far too little about how whole foods and the variety of nutrients they contain, impact the brain. However, it seems evident to me that the savoury, satisfying umami flavours that Buddhist monks developed to make plant-based foods more appealing also have a social quality. Popular foods such as pizza, spaghetti Bolognese, Thai curries, ramen, sushi and nasi goreng – which are tied to people's childhood memories around the world, fostering global cohesion – all pack a serious punch of umami flavour.

Eggs are especially rich in umami flavour. Eggs are often the first food that children learn to cook themselves. They are also a pagan symbol of the Christian festival of Easter, demonstrating that multiple traditions can come together as one. Eggs feature in festive customs like Easter egg tapping, which is popular across the German-speaking world and, elsewhere, goes by a host of different names, such as egg knocking and egg pacqueing. One player starts by hitting the tip of his opponent's egg with the tip of his egg, aiming to break the shell of his opponent's egg. Whoever's egg comes out unscathed wins. In German-speaking families, this game is played around the table on Easter morning. It's an old tradition and a striking example of how food is not simply nourishment but also has social and symbolic meaning.

The Chilean writer Isabel Allende's autobiographical book on the erotic joys of food describes a reconciliation ritual which features different ways of using umami.[9] After a fight with her husband, Allende makes a soup that is full of umami flavours. She uses chopped Portobello mushrooms, chopped porcino mushrooms, brown mushrooms, garlic, truffled olive oil, Port, vegetable stock, pepper, sour cream and a generous pinch of salt. Instead of adding all the Port and the olive oil to the dish, she keeps a few drops back and dabs them behind her ears as an aphrodisiac. She blends the ingredients in a mixer and simmers until the soup thickens and takes on a mouthwatering fragrance, awakening other secretions in both body and soul. Then she puts on her best dress, paints her fingernails red and serves her husband the soup in a pre-warmed bowl, garnished with a dollop of sour cream.

Hoping to experience the unifying power of flavour for myself, I conducted my own experiment by testing fifty different scents and recording how much each of them reminded me of social, communal experiences or moments of solitude. To my surprise, almost all the social scents were sweet (not exactly a diet I would recommend): toasted bread, roast hazelnuts, roast almonds, biscuits, caramel, coffee and butter. Ginger, black pepper, coconut, grass, dried figs, mint and apples prompted the least social feelings, even though I love all these flavours. The experiment showed me that I had introverted flavours, such as the scent of grass, which pulled me into my inner world and nature and extroverted ones, mainly the scents of toasting and baking, which transported me to my parents' house and more social environments. These social scents are not products of nature but new compounds which emerge through prolonged, careful exposure to heat. The fact that they predominantly occur in sweet foods – at least in my case – may have something to do with the fact that sugar activates the brain's reward system like no other nutrient. Either way, the experiment deepened my understanding of people who love sweet things, or who give them to their children. At this point, it is important to stress that just smelling these scents can evoke pleasant feelings of belonging; eating them is not necessary. On my daughter's birthdays, even unwrapping sweets proves itself to be of great social value, prompting fits of giggles and laughter. This shared sense of joy illustrates that the social value of these moments is not necessarily in eating them, but in imagining doing so.

As I mentioned previously, sour and bitter flavours can set off alarm signals that make us fear we are being poisoned. Even so, these flavours can also foster togetherness, particularly if they are bound up with a national or spiritual tradition. In South America, some tribespeople have a tradition of communally preparing bitter mate tea in a calabash. The host is first to drink the infusion of mate leaves in hot water, because it often tastes very bitter. This demonstrates his fortitude, which inspires the group to tolerate and enjoy the bitterness. In South Korea, kimchi, an aromatic, fermented condiment made from Chinese cabbage and other ingredients such as garlic, ginger, chilli powder and fish sauce, is a key part of the culture and national identity. It is served alongside practically every meal, whether with rice or as an ingredient in dishes such as kimchi pancakes, kimchi soup, or kimchi fried rice. People often make kimchi together in groups, with families and neighbours joining forces to prepare large quantities for winter. This practice fosters social connections and cohesion. The practice of consuming bitter herbs such as chicory, dandelion, endive and romaine lettuce during Passover is deeply embedded in the Jewish tradition. The bitter flavours commemorate the bitterness and suffering that their ancestors experienced during their enslavement in Egypt. This tradition can be understood both as an exercise in resilience and as a reminder that freedom can only be achieved in unison.

There is a unifying quality to the practice of sharing dishes. In Arab, African and Asian cultures, it is common to have many dishes on the table at once and for guests to partake of them all. This kind of communal eating reflects the importance of family, generosity and hospitality. It also helps expand one's taste horizons. It makes it much easier to consume the thirty different plant species we need to eat, as we learned in the previous chapter on the importance of diversity in food.

The generosity of cooking

For many people – including me – cooking is an exercise in resilience. What do my guests like? What do they hate? And what could go wrong? Too much salt, too much heat, too much sugar – and not out of neglect, but because of an excess of commitment and care. Cooking almost always involves generosity, intimacy and love that is looking for somewhere to go. What's more, dinner guests intuitively evaluate dishes with their mouths, their noses and their guts, so there's only a certain extent to which their response will be filtered and tempered. However, it is precisely this vulnerability, which every cook is familiar with, that is a foundation for deeper social bonds and friendships. This is why cooking and eating together are perfect ways to make new friends and tend to old friendships.

Fasting together can also strengthen bonds, whether through experiencing one's own limits as a group or through a shared desire for a new beginning. Almost all spiritual traditions have shared fasting days or periods that aid social cohesion and foster solidarity, because they remind those fasting that community always entails a degree of forgoing one's personal needs and naturally involves self-sacrifice.

The role of scent in mediating spiritual relationships

Scents play an important role in many spiritual traditions and practices and are often used to achieve spiritual experiences and expand consciousness. We have no real language for scents and usually have to reach for rough comparisons instead. Take, for instance, the phrase 'it smells like burning'. The complexity and intangibility of scent can foster a higher state of awareness. Smoked tree resins, such as frankincense and myrrh and the warm, woody fragrance of sandalwood are frequently used in church services and rituals to foster a sense of connection to the spiritual world.

But why are these woody scents of particular spiritual significance? Across the world, sacrificial rites were once at the heart of spiritual life, with meat and other foods being cooked over flames. For our ancestors, gathering around the fire and roasting a large, dead animal was a deeply emotive act, charged with divine significance. As such, it is fair to assume that spirituality was once closely tied to the experience of breathing in the smoky scent of barbecued meat. Even in the earliest Indian rituals, the smell of a fire was believed to placate the gods and invite them to the human dinner table, where they could partake of grilled foods alongside the people. As unpredictable and powerful as the gods were, Indian priests never once doubted that they shared humanity's weakness for the scent of grilled foods. Similarly, the advent of Judeo-Christian culture was accompanied by a host of smoky smells. Leviticus 3:5 states: "Then Aaron's sons are to burn it on the altar on top of the burnt offering that is lying on the burning wood; it is a food offering, an aroma pleasing to the Lord.' The ancient Hebrews had a different understanding of how God experienced scent. In Hebrew, the words for 'nose' and 'anger' have the same root. There was every possibility that the wrong kind of smoke might get up God's nose and provoke a snort of fury.[10]

As spirituality developed, the original smells of grilled meats were superseded by the smoky fragrance of burnt plants. In North America, a ceremonial pipe (known as a 'peace pipe' to colonial Europeans) was used by the Lakota, Cheyenne and Pawnee people to foster social and spiritual connections and resolve conflict. Tobacco was popular because its relaxing and mood-lifting effects were accompanied by smoke that made pleasant shapes, rising skyward and confirming the spiritual dimension of the peace it promised. Alongside tobacco, bearberries, mullein, lavender, sage, peppermint and juniper berries were also 'sacrificed' in the pipe bowl. In European antiquity, smoke from tree resins replaced animal sacrifices once used to commune with higher powers. Similarly, on the Day of the Dead, people in Mexico use the scent of freshly baked bread to make contact with their late ancestors. The altar is decked out with flowers, a cross, a picture of the deceased, baked goods, cobs of corn, fruit, incense and sweet-smelling bread. The scent of the bread is believed to tempt the ancestors back for a time to sit down with the living.

Similarly, in every religion where not only other-worldly spheres but certain people, living or dead, have been believed to exude spiritual powers, human bodily odour has been actively cultivated. The Ancient Egyptians developed methods for embalming their dead, aiming to transform them into immortal gods. New studies suggest that the Egyptians engaged in international trade, in part, to obtain the finest fragrances to make it more pleasant to commune with their divine ancestors. One key balsam, known by the Egyptian name 'antiu', did not contain myrrh or frankincense as was previously thought; it was actually a blend of cedar and cypress oil. There were special balms for each organ. Pistachio resin and castor oil were used exclusively for embalming the head; juniper was used for the liver and milk fat and beeswax ensured that the skin would retain eternal beauty.[11]

In Indian tradition, body odour was believed to reveal a person's karma. The Buddha is believed to have smelled like sandalwood, which is known for its soothing, cooling effects. This woody scent is part of a worldwide tradition of communal grilling, which has been refined in the West to become an offering of pure smoke. In Buddhism, fire takes a back seat. The Buddha, the great spiritual genius, transformed sacrificial rites into a series of mental processes. Yet he remained faithful to that woody scent, because it hints at the origins of connectedness in a way that no other sensory stimulus can.

In Christianity, the Son of God smells like bread and is responsible for ensuring that the pleasant scent of eternal life reaches every corner of the world. This is strikingly clear in the story of the raising of Lazarus, who was dead for four days and who, the Bible says, stank terribly. With his spiritual gifts, Jesus transformed the stench of death into the fragrance of life. In gratitude, Lazarus' sister Maria anointed Jesus with a pound of nard, a priceless, aromatic oil. She used so much of the oil that she had to dry Jesus's feet with her own hair, which saw her enter into a kind of fragrance-based communion with him. The disciples were appalled, 'Why this waste?' they cried, 'You could have sold the oil and given the money to the poor!' Yet Jesus points to their moment of fragrant, spiritual communion and tells them that, by anointing him with oil, the woman has prepared him for burial. Anointing with oil is so central to Christianity that Jesus himself was given the names Christ and Messiah, both of which stem from the Hebrew verb for 'to anoint'. After Jesus's death on the cross, the stench of death never came, replaced instead by a wonderful, calming fragrance. The scent itself was just one indication that Jesus was the Son of God.

I decided to perform a series of personal experiments to gauge the spiritual potential of smoky and woody scents. A friend of mine who teaches Catholicism gave me the necessary tools to experiment with frankincense: sand, coal and some frankincense – little balls of yellow, red, black and white resin. Following her instructions, I scattered the sand on the bottom of the incense burner, then used a pair of tongs to hold the piece of coal and light it with a match. It sent out a spray of yellow and orange sparks. I set it down on top of the sand and waited for it to turn grey. I then scattered a little sand on top, followed by the colourful resin balls. I was surprised by how lovely the smoke looked as it rose from the burner. It smelt like fire and the glowing coal reminded me of the first burnt offerings. The smoke was rich with sweet, balsamic, aromatic and lemony notes, which gave it an air of mysticism. Was this a sign of a higher power, one that burned and renewed life, enriching it with unfathomable depths and secrets, leading it to places that went beyond language? The smoke soon filled my entire living room, seeping into every corner. I had been hoping for an intimate experience, but it never materialised. Instead, the incense had inspired a kind of awe in me, sending my focus outwards and onto bigger things. I saw the great altar of Pergamon with its relief depicting the Gigantomachy, which I had admired so much in Berlin. I saw the mighty columns of smoke rising proudly skyward from Abel's sacrificial offering, kindling Cain's murderous jealousy. I saw inside the cupolas of the Sistine Chapel and beheld Noah's family watching over the sacrificial fire, offering two rams. The scent of the incense revealed to me its original, social character. It seemed better suited to intimate self-reflection than to grand festivities and mystic cults. It called to mind images of a great congregation hoping to honour and appease a short-tempered god with marble altars, impressive reliefs, majestic columns of smoke and grand sacrifices of rams.

For my second experiment, I used a braid of American sweetgrass, given to me by a friend who had spent many years in the US studying shamanism. For my friend, the grass represented Mother Earth's fragrant hair. Indeed, it smelt like black earth, but also like river water, honey and vanilla. The scent of sweetgrass can evoke experiences and memories we often haven't even realised we have forgotten. Sweetgrass smoke is believed to cleanse the aura and is used to conjure benevolent spirits. I set about burning one end of the braid of grass. It gave off a pleasantly aromatic, sweet scent. Breathing it in, I felt a strong sense of connection with nature. Its woody notes reminded me of the campfire I had sat around as a boy scout. And then, in the background, I could hear shamanic drumming and voices singing a song that I had learned on a course about North American shamanism: 'Hey hey hey, Wakan Tanka, hey hey hey'. I entered into a mild trance, stepping into another time, one that was not linear but cyclical. While I was in this state, everything slipped away from me, then came flooding back, all of it rolling on like a wheel. Everything died, everything blossomed again, everything said its farewells, everything came back and said hello and remained true to itself forever. The centre of time was everywhere and I could feel it, here and now, in the burning hair of Mother Earth.

For my third experiment into the spirituality of scent, I wanted to experience the karmic fragrance of sandalwood. A friend of mine works in a perfumery and recommended that I use perfumes for my experiment, because, to this day, some of the most expensive and mysterious perfumes smell like sandalwood, which is known as 'santal' in French. She gave me a few small test bottles: Santal by Guerlain, Santal Blanc by Van Cleef & Arpels, White Sandalwood by Goldfield & Banks, Molecule 04 by Escentric Molecules and Most Wanted by Azzaro. All the fragrances were cooling and calming. The cheapest sandalwood fragrance, from Azzaro, contained the fewest secrets. Its name, 'Most Wanted', said it loud and clear: like a campfire or a ritual bonfire, its woody scent was intended to kindle people's energies and bind them together. The scent was pleasant, but I felt that it was too flat and too likeable for my spiritual experiment. The sandalwood from Guerlain seemed too feminine for my purposes and the Australian one from Goldfield & Banks was much too masculine. My friend advised that Escentric Molecules perfumes were subtle and likely to be picked up on unconsciously. The 04 fragrance is pure sandalwood. I did find that I didn't consciously smell it, but it seemed to relax me and created a sense of connectedness. Yet its subtlety was likewise unsuitable for my experiment. Ultimately, I opted for Santal Blanc by Van Cleef & Arpels; it smelled like a distillation of the soothing, unifying effect of a campfire.

At home, I sprayed my bedroom with Santal Blanc. My children had spent the duration of my incense experiment worrying about the risks of a housefire and had turned their noses up at the smoke from my shamanistic sweetgrass, claiming it was 'too strong'.

Now, they were sniffing the air eagerly. Later that night, once I had put them to bed, I took a sniff straight from the bottle, but unfortunately, no visions appeared before my eyes. I decided to carry out another, more intensive sandalwood experiment another day. I used the incense burner, the sand and the coal that I had used for the frankincense experiment, but this time, I burned sandalwood shavings. I also put a little finely ground sandalwood on my tongue. Powdered sandalwood is sold as a spice and a baking dye. I sniffed a cloth I had sprayed with Santal Blanc. All this combined to create an extremely intense scent that brought a vision to mind: I was standing around a fire with other people, cloaked in animal furs and breathing in the smell of a roasting bull's leg, as droplets of liquid fat dripped from the meat and sizzled in the flames. We were singing and looking up at the starry sky, confident in the knowledge that we were not alone in the world. And then, the furs transformed into fine clothes, pleasantly soft and an old man, most likely a Brahmin, was singing a strange-sounding chant, ending on an 'Om'. A second older man arrived, sporting a long beard and wrinkled his nose. You could see that the smell of our meat cooking had bothered him. Next, the fire went out and the meat disappeared. We were standing around the campfire sheepishly, scattering warm ash on our heads. This induced a brief frenzy, in which I lost any sense of time or place. When I awoke from it, I was standing in a monastery in front of a statue of the Buddha that smelled strongly of sandalwood. The monks were laughing away merrily, even though there was nothing to laugh about. I laughed heartily along with them. In the background, I could hear a singing bowl. I found myself sitting at a great table with many other people. A young man with long hair was talking. The mood was grave. He broke off a piece of fragrant bread, fresh from a wood-fired oven, and spoke words that were somehow meaningful yet paradoxical all at once. Each of us placed the piece of bread we received on our tongues. It tasted terrific, like wood and hot coals. The man called on us to eat the bread slowly and with grace, because the bread was him. He was the bread of life and the scent of life. And then, all of a sudden, I was a young man in the US, feeling lonely. Someone waved me over, shouting, 'Barbecue! Do you want to join?' I nodded and followed him. He proudly selected a juicy steak from the grill and put it on my plate. It smelled fantastic. His wife and kids smiled at me. In broad American accents edged with excitement, they told me the story of a cowboy who wins a barbecue cook-off. I could only partly understand their enthusiasm, but it felt like I had belonged to that community of scents and flavours forever.

After that, I lay down on my bed and soon fell asleep. It was profoundly moving to experience the effects of this fragrance firsthand. It evoked memories of experiences that I explored in my book, *Higher Self.*

The power of alcohol to bring us together

I would be guilty of a serious omission if I tried to write a chapter about communal eating without looking into the impact of alcohol. Alcohol was performing essential social and spiritual functions, such as facilitating access to other people, or making contact with one's ancestors or gods, for millennia before Jesus used wine to convince people of the divine nature of communion.

Digesting alcohol poses a significant challenge for our bodies. A full ten per cent of the countless enzymes in our livers are devoted to breaking down alcohol. Despite this outlay, however, our capacity to break down alcohol is limited, such that large quantities of alcohol can damage our liver, heart and brain. There is a theory that our relatively good capacity to digest small amounts of alcohol has granted us a decisive evolutionary advantage, enabling us to access longer-lasting, non-perishable calories. However, there was a different social aspect to alcohol consumption. Since drunkenness could lead to people having minor accidents, getting lost, or falling prey to predators, human beings had to band together to protect each other when they were drunk. Even chimpanzees who have access to alcohol rarely drink it alone, instead choosing to do so in company.

The rituals of the Camba people in eastern Bolivia attest to the importance of alcohol in fostering togetherness between human beings.[12] The Camba people are genetically less capable of digesting alcohol; just a few sips and they feel dizzy and ready to throw up. Despite this, they drink high-proof rum during rituals, because it boosts a sense of belonging – and they are happy to accept the physical consequences in return.

Alcohol provokes an intense release of dopamine, making drinkers extra sociable. It also prompts the body to release GABA, the brain's key soothing messenger, which suppresses social anxiety and inhibitions. Stimulating the endorphin system with alcohol causes us to forget physical and psychological pain, leading to greater affirmation of other people and their opinions and of ourselves. There is a kind of mysticism in saying yes to life unconditionally, as opposed to sober-mindedness, which evaluates, judges, divides and separates.

Unfortunately, however, the effects of alcohol are not always prosocial and can also have the opposite impact. Alcohol can make us generous and talkative, but it can also make us disinterested and indifferent; it can make us feel loved up, but jealous and irritable; quick-witted, but brainless too. Alcohol can stimulate our hearts and minds and yet it also causes lasting damage to these organs. This is why consuming alcohol not only enhances social rituals but also *requires* rituals to limit the quantity and speed at which it is consumed, to steer those unfettered mental energies in a positive direction. Human beings' dealings with alcohol have taught us that we need the self-restraint and rituals that spirituality provides to tap into and realise our own social and mystic potential. It's no coincidence that Sister André, a spiritual expert in longevity, indulged in a glass of wine at lunch every day with her fellow residents.

Transforming Nutritional Energy

In this chapter, I want to expand on mindful eating by examining the energy the food we eat transforms into in our bodies. Claudia, whom I mentioned in the introduction, was not capable of converting the artificial food she was taking in into a life-giving stream of energy in the long term, which is why she sadly died at such a young age. Esther, whom we met in the previous chapter, struggled to turn nutritional energy into interpersonal energy. By contrast, Kane Tanaka, Sister André and Grandma Anna succeeded in mindfully transforming the food they ate into physical, social and spiritual energy, as evidenced by the great ages they reached, their sense of gratitude and their devotion to fellow human beings.

When I say energy here, I mean both objective bodily energies and the energy that we subjectively sense and intuit. The body's energy budget is essentially governed by the limbic system, particularly the hypothalamus. This tiny but crucial part of the brain has direct contact with sensory nerves and nutrients in the cerebrospinal fluid, which enable it to respond quickly to diet, environmental changes and emotional perceptions. It employs neuropeptides to influence other parts of the brain, such as the limbic system, which is responsible for emotions. It can regulate energy flow throughout the body via hormones, the vagus nerve and the sympathetic nervous system. This is particularly evident in cases of acute stress: the body reacts to a threatening dog by expending more energy, which manifests as anxiety, feeling hot, a raised pulse, or sweating.

Scholars in Asia had suspicions about the existence of this energy system as far back as three thousand years ago. They were very familiar with animal anatomy and developed meditation techniques that enabled them to sense and visualise streams of energy within the body. They understood that there were important energy centres connected to the spinal cord and they named these 'chakras', meaning 'wheel' or 'disc' in Sanskrit. Chakras can open or close like flowers – a good image for how the hormonal glands work, as they are activated or deactivated by chemical signals from the hypothalamus. These glands include the thyroid, adrenal glands, ovaries and testicles, which are assigned to the throat chakra, the abdominal chakra and the sacral chakra, respectively. However, the chakras also correspond to the nerve plexuses to which the vagus nerve and the sympathetic nervous system are connected and which are arranged along the spinal column. The largest plexus, the solar plexus, is assigned to the navel chakra, which is responsible for digestion. According to the Indian concept, chakras are tasked with transforming energy, such as converting energy from food into sexual or social energy. They are connected via channels known as 'nadi' in Sanskrit, which literally translates as 'tube', 'nerve', or 'pulse'. Scholars believed there were 350,000 nadis in our bodies, which they believed corresponded to the nervous system. They identified one major channel and two secondary channels. All three of these were thought to run along the spinal column and the major channel was believed to pass directly through the chakras, which correspond to the nerve connections between the nerve plexuses along the spinal cord. The secondary channels were thought to lie to the left and right of this, representing the two streams of hormones, analogous to the anatomical fact that hormonal glands form pairs: there are sex glands and hormonal glands located on both sides of the body, while the thyroid gland and thymus are each composed of a left and right lobe. In Indian philosophy, it is believed that there is no circulation in these channels, which contradicts the understanding of the nadis as blood vessels. Instead, the streams of nutrients flow in one direction, the way water flows from the roots of a tree to its crown, or like wind driving rain clouds across a field. The oldest Eastern concepts of bodily energies come from Indian midwives, who used the flow of nutrients from mother to child via the umbilical cord as a basis for understanding the flow of energies in relationships.

For centuries, the concept of chakras and nadis served to explain how the body functions. The energy flowing through this system is known as prana in India and qi in China, where healing techniques such as acupuncture were developed based on these teachings. The concept of energy helped people understand the connection between metabolism and consciousness and to create a psychology of impulses, emotions and motivations. The idea of 'tantra' emerged over the course of this process and encompasses much more than sexuality. Tantric teaching, which exerted a significant influenced on all Eastern traditions, including Buddhism and Hinduism, proceeds on the assumption that impurities and blockages in the chakras and nadis cause illnesses and hamper wellbeing and that healing techniques such as acupuncture, acupressure, shiatsu, Tai Chi and tantric sexual practices can provide the opportunity to resolve these blockages in the flow of energy, thereby improving both mental and physical wellbeing.

These teachings on energy not only prompted the development of powerful healing techniques but also contributed to the growth of Eastern spirituality. Much like in the West, the early days of Indian thinking were dominated by the notion that body and mind were strictly separate. However, unlike in the West, the two-worlds teaching was criticised much earlier in India, because it contradicted the Eastern understanding of wholeness and unity. For centuries, scholars have sought a solution to this dilemma. The *Bhagavad Gita*, a key work of Hindu scripture which brings together different schools of thought, solved the problem of body vs soul by embracing a nourishing energy that unites all things. The God of sustenance stands for the sanctity of life, for the powerful, unshakeable conclusion that the One always also refers to the dyad of body and mind. In the *Bhagavad Gita*, the God of sustenance declares: 'I am both the life force and the stuff of life, both at once.'[1]

Every day, food offers us the opportunity to experience this interconnected duality for ourselves, as food and as vital energy.

These Eastern teachings are often misunderstood in the West because Western philosophy has established such a stark separation between matter and spirit that the energies of the chakras and nadis are understood purely in spiritual terms. In the Indian tradition, the spiritual or 'subtle' aspect of this teaching concerns consciously experiencing and visualising energies and their influence, but these energies are not purely spiritual; they relate to our physical bodies and the food we eat. Over time, however, affinities have developed between the Eastern and Western traditions. The Greek athletic ideal embodies a similar ethos, which holds that physical fitness is the prerequisite for moral, personal and intellectual development. It's a concept that lives on in modern physical education classes. In Christianity, the energetic, ethereal nature of bread and wine is at the heart of the Last Supper. Judaism and Islam have established mystical traditions which see nutritional energies transform into gaseous, ascending spiritual energies. Modern Western depth psychology also encompasses some of Eastern thinking's fundamental ideas on energy. When Sigmund Freud or Carl Jung speak about the libido or the life force being blocked, fixated, repelled, split, or repressed, they are adopting the Indian concept of energy, be it consciously or unconsciously. Meanwhile, this holistic view is exerting an increasing influence on the neurosciences. On 9 November 2023, the date of writing, the natural sciences journal *Nature* published an editorial titled, 'Brain and body are more intertwined than we knew'. It is a call to neuroscientists to look beyond the brain to the body as a whole and to clinicians who work with the body, inviting them to keep the body's connections to the brain in mind. The new scientific fields of psychoendocrinology, stress research, psychoneuroimmunology, epigenetics and neuroplasticity all deal with the connection between consciousness, the mind and the body.

The field of psychoneuroimmunology offers a contemporary example of the importance of the physical energy system to our well-being. Autonomic dysregulation can result from a COVID-19 infection and is a disorder of the autonomic nervous system, which comprises the vagus nerve and the sympathetic nervous system. Antibodies can be a cause of this, damaging the nervous system by triggering an autoimmune response. One sign that the system is malfunctioning is a profound and lasting drop in blood pressure when getting up after sleeping, which manifests as dizziness. All parts of the autonomic nervous system are affected, leading to many debilitating symptoms, from breathlessness, chest pain, palpitations, tiredness and physical exhaustion with no apparent cause, anxiety, to digestive complaints and diarrhoea. These symptoms can last for weeks or even longer after a mild illness; those affected experience firsthand what happens when the body's energy is not optimally converted and distributed. Fortunately, the damage almost always recedes over a period of weeks to months.

In the section below, I hope to use the teaching on the chakras to shed light on the energy system and demonstrate how we can influence it through visualisations, exercise and diet. The scientific basis for the energy system lies in the hypothalamus, which sits directly beneath the thalamus, the gateway to perception, immediately behind the optic nerves' intersection. Its interconnected position in the brain suggests we could alter the body's energy balance through targeted awareness, meditation and energy visualisations. In practical terms, I am interested in expanding on mindful and conscious eating by experiencing the nutritional energy and the nutrient flows into which the food we eat is transformed. This is why I find myself reaching both for the Eastern traditions and the teachings of Hildegard von Bingen. Hildegard was convinced that human beings should not sleep or otherwise distract themselves after eating; she believed they should maintain a degree of awareness until the taste, the juices and the scent of the food they had consumed reached the proper place. If not, Hildegard argued, these might end up in the wrong place, blown this way and that like dust on the wind.

The naval chakra (digestive energy)

Medically speaking, you might compare the storage and transformation of nutritional energy to a small fridge kept in a flat and a big chest freezer kept in the cellar. Energy derived from food is primarily stored as sugar chains in the liver (or fridge) and, once this is full, it is transferred to the cellar, where it is stored as fat. By the same token, energy is only brought up out of the chest freezer in the basement when the fridge in the flat is almost empty. The hormone insulin plays a significant role in this decision. When there is a lot of insulin in our blood, it is unlikely we will go down to the cellar to pick up more energy, because insulin signals that the stores are full. Thus, we find ourselves using more energy to go down to the basement. Low insulin levels, whether they be provoked by fasting or a low-carbohydrate diet, can tap the vast energy stores in fatty tissue. This explains the paradoxical experience that sees people forgoing calories exhibiting a boost in physical energy and people with high blood sugar due to a metabolic condition often suffering from anxiety, a lack of energy and daytime drowsiness.

Alongside insulin, which responds to snacks and sugary food, the stress hormones governed by the hypothalamus are also responsible for shutting the chest freezer in the cellar. This is why people under stress have less energy and tend to develop abdominal fat. In cases of persistent stress, the body only feeds from the small fridge in the flat, giving rise to the false impression that the fridge comprises our total energy potential. People experiencing burnout will occasionally remember that they have significant stores in the cellar, but stress will soon make them forget about them again. For many people suffering from stress, it takes a crisis, a radical lifestyle change, severe hardship, or some journey to send them back to the cellar. Practising relaxation through meditation, breathing techniques and yoga can help us avoid losing touch with the energetic potential in the basement (i.e., fat stores).

The storage and transformation of energy from food is visualised as the navel chakra. This chakra is yellow, like fire, representing the metabolism and the burning process of transformation. It also includes the ideal transformation and preparation of nutritional energy through cooking, as well as the destruction of nutritional energy caused by industrial overheating. This chakra is compared to the roots of a tree, storing and delivering energy. Trees are of great spiritual significance in the Eastern tradition – after all, the Buddha achieved enlightenment under a tree – so it is no surprise that Eastern scholars visualise the body's flows of energy as a tree. In the old Ayurvedic texts, the gut corresponds to the roots and the trunk of the tree, from which the internal organs sprout like branches, corresponds to the liver, the gallbladder and the pancreas. What is interesting is that it aligns reasonably well with both modern evolutionary teaching and modern embryology. In the beginning was the Gut.

The navel chakra sits level with the navel, directly in front of the spinal column at the point where the solar plexus and the pancreas are located, the latter providing insulin, which is essential for regulating nutritional energy. From today's perspective, it would make sense to include the enteric nervous system in this chakra. The enteric nervous system has over five hundred million nerve cells, more than twice as many as the bone marrow and the autonomic nervous system and almost as many as an adult cat. The enteric nervous system responds to food independently of the brain. It makes energetically important decisions on blood distribution, muscle activity, the release of digestive juices and immune defence, as well as consciously perceiving and experiencing digestion itself. A stomach ache reminds us that the body's first nervous system evolved in the gut and that our earliest ancestors were little more than tubular creatures whose only response to the world was to contract to escape potential harm. This intestinal consciousness lives on in us.

Although human beings have a sophisticated enteric nervous system, our guts are decidedly small when compared to our brains. We are like enormous trees with tiny roots, naturally inclined to be top-heavy. Furthermore, the enteric nervous system can operate autonomously, which increases the risk of emotional disconnection from nutritional energy. An inability to sense the energy we get from our food often leads to a lack of satiety and overeating. Conversely, a stronger sense of mental rootedness in the navel chakra can reduce calorie intake and improve energy balance.

According to Eastern scholars, blockages in the flows of energy and energy build-up in a chakra can impact personality. In the chakra teachings, an organism's ability to retain and manage nutritional energy in the abdomen is a sign of power. This is why the navel chakra's energy is characterised by willpower and perseverance. However, when this chakra is dominant, it is comparable to a state with significant oil reserves whose policies predominantly focus on distributing the income from oil sales to a small group of privileged people, to the detriment of the country as a whole. By contrast, people with a weak navel chakra are weak-willed, lacking focus and self-restraint. They are completely disconnected from the oil reserves. The Latin word *focus* – meaning hearth or fireplace – can help us intuitively understand this teaching. Having a focus in life means having a fire onto which we consciously project and concentrate energy and which can be converted into drive and goal orientation. A lack of access to a metabolic inner fire of this kind leads to an inability to consciously enjoy the beneficial and rewarding arrival of nutritional energy after a meal, which can contribute to binge eating, overeating and obesity. If I am feeling hungry, passive and unable to focus on a task, I like to pay close attention to my stomach, as this helps me realise I am not making the most of my energy at that moment. I then want to say to my stomach, 'Unlock your potential!' This works like a mantra, helping me to find new energy.

Mindful eating is the simplest and best way to connect with the nutritional energy in our abdomens. According to Indian teaching, controlled abdominal breathing can encourage the flow of nutritional energies both during and after eating. When stress limits your ability to tune into your gut activity, it can help to place both hands on your belly and consciously feel its curvature as you breathe. I've observed that visualising flames and yellow energy can help to stimulate my own digestion. In the

Ayurvedic tradition, yellow foods such as corn, bananas and turmeric are believed to benefit the navel chakra. Yoga poses that strengthen the abdominal muscles, such as the boat and butterfly poses and Pilates exercises that centre the body, are believed to do the same. A succession of yoga poses similar to a sun salutation can help to distribute the energy from the navel chakra throughout the body. All these methods have their limits, however. Take Claudia, for instance. Her gut was not functioning as it should have, meaning that nutritional energy was not being properly digested and these energy exercises alone would not have been able to save her.

The sacral chakra (vital energy)

The sacral chakra is located directly underneath the navel chakra. According to the Indian tradition, the sacral chakra converts nutritional energy into an all-round zest for life that includes sensuality and sexuality but also goes beyond these – it is the very foundation for taking an interest in the world. According to Freud, in the first year of our lives – the oral phase – we learn to expand our desire for food into a more general lust for life. In this case, the term 'oral' indicates that for an infant, the mouth is the primary source of gratification, i.e. through suckling and nursing. The infant discovers that the nourishing energy of its mother's milk also resonates with a sense of joy at being at the breast, which then gradually extends to include the mother as a whole and her environment. During this phase, we learn to understand our existence as pleasurable; we know that life is worth living. Freud's theory is based on observing that in periods of severe stress and profound uncertainty, our lust for life decreases and our oral needs increase, be that a need for pure calories, cigarettes, or the urge to bite our nails. These oral cravings can manifest later in life as depression. The theory of the oral phase is also interesting from the perspective of evolutionary biology because the first larger groups of intestinal nerve cells formed at the anterior opening of the primitive gut – i.e., the primitive mouth – from which our brains ultimately developed, together with all their functions and interests.

The sacral chakra is located in the lower abdomen, around two fingers' width below the belly button. Deep below this sits the nerve plexus, which governs the sexual organs. Breathing into the abdomen can help to strengthen this chakra. The sacral chakra's energy is believed to be orange, with an appropriate visualisation being a pulsing orange ball. Mantras such as 'My emotions flow freely' and 'I am in touch with my creativity' can help us connect to the sacral chakra. Yoga positions such as warrior II, butterfly pose, or fish pose can help to balance sacral energy. Ayurveda recommends orange foods such as oranges, mangoes, carrots and sweet potatoes, as well as essential oils with citrus and orange scents, to help foster sacral creativity. Taking a relaxing bath or meditating in water can also activate this chakra because it is connected to the water element. Creative activities such as painting, writing, dancing, or playing music, as well as interacting with works of art, can also help balance sacral chakra energy.

The root chakra (groundedness and material security)

The root chakra sits at the base of the spinal column, near the coccyx. Its original Sanskrit name is Muladhara, which literally means 'root support'. It is dark red in colour and associated with the earth element. Its energy connects the body to the Earth and to the physical world. In Freud's theory of development, this chakra corresponds to the anal stage, where control over one's stool takes prominence. The coccygeal plexus is responsible for this, governing the rectum, intestinal blockages and defecation.

Freud ascribed a significant role to the rectum in his teachings. He worked on the premise that a child's anal phase lasts from when they are eighteen months to the age of three. According to Freud, the practical development tasks that a child undertakes during this time include learning and strengthening their ability to control excretion. A child's stool is the first thing that the child produces themselves, which can either give or refuse to its parents, which, Freud claims, is a precursor to dealing with money and power. According to Freud, the influence this period has on a child's personality depends on whether the parents give the child free rein and allow them to soil themselves, are sensitive in helping them deal with their stool, or are forceful in taking it away. According to this theory, excessive focus on control can lead to an anal fixation, which manifests as stubbornness, a love of tidiness, or a desire for control. If parents are too lax in their approach, it can lead to a chaotic lifestyle, instability, waste and financial problems.

The theory of the anal stage is not scientific. Still, the notion of an anal person who loves order, punctuality, cleanliness, precision and an eye for financial and material matters has persisted. It is also interesting to note that Indian teaching ascribes the same psychic qualities to the gut, specifically security and a stable material existence. In contrast to Freud, it places less emphasis on childhood and more on the lifelong task of nourishing and tending to the root chakra. A healthy root chakra is associated with security, being well grounded and a feeling of belonging. Anxiety and stress are typical disruptors of root energy. If a person is dealt a blow and braces internally, the openings to their body, including the mouth and the anus, naturally contract. Their breathing turns shallow. Fittingly, the word 'Angst' or 'anxiety' in German originally meant 'narrow' or 'narrowing'. Thus, we detach ourselves, piece by piece, from the vital energy that flows through us via the food we eat and our breath. This may make sense in the short term, but if this reaction becomes a regular or lasting occurrence, it generates a feeling of alienation, torpor and a loss of energy. The Taoist tradition holds that blocked energies in the root chakra cannot flow through the main channels, leading them to seek alternative side channels or to leak out, which can manifest as involuntary movements and sensations in the body, such as pain, itching, feeling cold, feeling hot, tinnitus and constipation.

In Indian tradition, a simple exercise to invigorate the root chakra involves clenching the anal sphincter for a few seconds before consciously relaxing it. This is followed by a single breath in and out through the mouth, helping open the entire digestive system and get the energy moving. When performing a root chakra meditation, it is also recommended that you concentrate on the tip of your nose. This may be because the part of the brain that represents the root chakra is connected to the nose. The nose is also level with the hypothalamus, which boosts awareness via the hormone hypocretin, which promotes wakefulness, helping the earthy root energies to bloom. The root chakra is directly connected to the sense of smell due to its association with the earth element. It's a matter of smelling what we and others want to smell. Helpful mantras for meditation might include phrases such as 'I am safe and protected', 'I trust life' and 'I am firmly rooted in the Earth'.

When it comes to feeding the root chakra, Ayurveda recommends root vegetables such as carrots, potatoes, parsnips, radishes, turnips, onions, garlic and protein-rich foods such as eggs, meat, beans, tofu, soya products and peanut butter. Suitable herbs and spices include chives, paprika and pepper. Ayurveda also suggests touching or carrying grounding crystals such as black onyx, reddish-brown hematite, or red jasper. These stones may help to invigorate and balance out the root chakra.

There is a particular spiritual dimension to the root chakra alongside its importance for energy and health.

In esoteric and spiritual traditions, primarily Hinduism and some yoga practices, the root chakra's spiritual potential is visualised as a serpent-like energy called Kundalini, which sleeps coiled at the base of the spine. The awakening and rising of Kundalini is understood as a process of cleansing and flooding all the chakras with energy, clearing blockages and allowing for spiritual growth and a deeper energy awareness. It is important to stress that this awakening can also have a dangerous side. If the energy that is released flows outside of the three channels, this can lead to a loss of grip on reality and the development of a psychotic state. All this shows that material security, self-control and social support are not obstacles to spiritual growth; in fact, they are essential to it.

The heart chakra (social energy)

Having discussed how the energy from the food we eat moves deep into the body to the centres of desire, power and groundedness, I now want to look more closely at the energy that rises from these centres into the heart. This ascent is of great importance in both Ayurvedic medicine and Eastern spirituality, yet the concept of experiencing the world with one's heart is also a Christian commandment.

According to Indian beliefs, there is a lot that can go wrong when nutritional energy ascends. The energy can distribute itself and dissipate across numerous side channels, feeding attractions, repulsions and illusions that, in turn, result in desire, greed, hate, envy and addiction. The more the body succeeds in opening up the central channel and transferring all the energy to the heart chakra, the greater the feeling of vigour, motivation, freedom, balance and compassion. This is precisely what the Tantric meditation, also known as the inner fire meditation, seeks to achieve: to bring the body's energies together in one central location and have them flow freely into the heart chakra, where they are transformed into more subtle, sincere energies.

According to Indian teaching, a blossoming heart chakra manifests as empathy, a capacity for love, social openness, emotional intelligence and spiritual feelings such as 'The whole world is within me,' 'I am within everything,' and 'Everything is connected.' In my experience, the loving-kindness meditation is particularly effective at transforming nutritional energy into love and goodwill towards oneself and others. First, you send loving thoughts to yourself, then to someone close to you, then to people you don't know well and eventually to the whole world. When you do this, you should pay attention to the wealth of energy that flows into your chest. It can also be helpful to repeat mantras such as 'I love and accept myself', 'I open my heart to love and compassion', aloud or quietly to yourself. Yoga exercises can also help to strengthen the heart chakra, such as warrior I, warrior II and camel pose. It can also help to spend time in nature, particularly in peaceful, relaxing places. Lastly, maintaining a loving and unselfish attitude towards others is always an exceptionally effective way to open your heart chakra and transform that nutritional energy into compassion.

The throat chakra (communication and speech)

In the Eastern tradition, the throat chakra is the energy centre associated with breathing, speaking, communication, creativity, authenticity and self-expression.

It includes the thyroid, which is governed by the hypothalamus and produces hormones which regulate the body's metabolism. Thyroid hormones are vital for normal growth and the development of tissue, organs and the nervous system. Biologically speaking, thyroid hormones can decrease body weight, increase motivation and elevate mood. This is why they are also used in psychiatry, where they have been found to boost the effects of antidepressants. Both Western and Eastern holistic medicines had associated the throat chakra with obesity long before the discovery of thyroid hormones. The Greek philosopher Aristotle observed that compulsive eaters exclusively experienced their food in their throats, which led to feelings of insatiability. The Hindu mystic Patanjali, who was responsible for shaping yoga teaching, also considered the throat to be a site of insatiability. He recommended the following mantra for withstanding hunger and thirst: 'Hunger pipe in the throat, dissolve!' Liquids such as water, herbal tea and clear soups also help to soothe the throat's cravings.

If the throat chakra is closed, nutritional energy can become stuck in the throat, preventing it from reaching the sacral and root chakras. Freud would argue that people experiencing this kind of blockage are orally fixated. An orally fixated person will struggle to find stability and stand on their own two feet. They cling to others and do not enjoy being alone. Occasionally, they will turn their backs on everything around them. Still, they are ultimately out for themselves because true closeness to others would only heighten their oral desire to an unbearable degree. They almost always feel a sense of emptiness because their food gets stuck and fails to satisfy them. They often have mood swings and episodes of depression and feel, not infrequently, that the world owes them something. Expressions such as 'mouthy' and 'mouthing off' are good descriptors of blocked throat energies. Possible consequences of blocked throat energies include cramping of the masticatory muscles and painful conditions of the jaw joint. Conversely, turning quiet and displaying a penchant for abstract, vague and negative thinking are signs that the throat chakra is not receiving enough energy.

Human beings feel at home not just in their bodies but also in language, so that communicative throat energies can be particularly valuable for health and well-being. They make it possible to convert feelings, sensations and experiences into language, to connect with oneself and to connect with other people. The intimate, intuitive language of mantras, poetry and song is particularly well-suited when it comes to making the throat chakra bloom. However, feelings which are not verbalised and recognised cannot be fully felt. 'I feel depressed', 'I feel excluded', 'I feel attacked', 'I feel ashamed', 'I feel unloved', 'I feel hopeless', 'I feel judged', 'I feel lonely' – all too often, feelings such as these are simply translated as 'I feel hungry'. This error in translation transforms them back into metabolic needs, making it impossible to learn from, grow from and process them.

The balancing effects of language are well documented across cultures. In Greek mythology, Poseidon's words have the power to calm the waves. In the Bible, Jesus walks on water and calms a storm with a word. Eastern spirituality has developed meditation techniques to strengthen the throat chakra. The Buddhist monk Thích Nhất Hạnh once said, 'A mindful breath is a good way for your body to 'snack' on some mindfulness and recognise and embrace strong feelings that may be there. After a mindful breath, you may have less desire to go and fill up on a snack to distract yourself. Your body is nourished by your breath.'[2]

For all the reasons above, it is important to express oneself clearly and authentically – breathing fully into the belly when speaking – and to communicate mindfully. Breathing exercises, singing and journaling can help boost these skills. The throat chakra is visualised as a pale blue, pulsating energy that spreads from the throat across the body. This image can be helpful for meditation, and you can support it by wearing blue clothing, stones and necklaces. Certain yoga poses can also help open the throat chakra, such as the bridge, fish and plough poses.

The third eye chakra (insight and wisdom)

The third eye chakra, also known as the Ajna, or brow chakra, is the centre of energy associated with perception, intuition, recognition, imagination and spiritual consciousness. It sits between the eyes, at the base of the nose, corresponding to the transition point between the thalamus, which coordinates perception and the hypothalamus, the energy centre. According to Indian teachings, the third eye chakra is the seat of wisdom, insight, imagination, intelligence and confidence. Essentially, it helps to keep an eye on things. With this in mind, we might say that scientists such as Albert Einstein, mystics like Hildegard von Bingen and psychiatrists such as Carl Jung exhibited signs of a blooming third eye chakra, enabling them to inject energy into their abstract physical, theological and psychological ideas and unite mind, body and matter. Artists such as Frida Kahlo and Picasso used their well-connected third-eye energy to transform their extraordinary powers of perception into artworks that have inspired generations ever since.

If the thalamus and hypothalamus do not communicate adequately, this can manifest as aloofness, which we might interpret as a sign of a closed third-eye chakra. Sufferers are typically blinded by expectations and fixed ideas and can become frustrated when the world and their peers fail to meet those expectations. Body and mind are separate. People with this character type tend to be indiscriminate, unbalanced, or chaotic in their eating habits and a portion of the nutritional energy they consume will not flow down through the body; instead, it moves upwards, unprocessed, prompting a split in thinking, feeling and bodily sensations. This can cause a person's thinking to become disconnected from the social world and material things, signalling an energetic withdrawal from the world and from the body. The person will avoid intimate, emotional relationships. In the body itself, this may manifest as a cold face, cold hands and cold feet. The person will rarely make eye contact. Facial muscles are often tense and the person's face appears mask-like. They are also likely to suffer from headaches and migraines. They will move through the world with meagre, flat feelings, yet as soon as their blocked energies find an outlet, they may be expressed explosively as rage and hostility. At best, their hypersensitivity and overly intellectual approach to the world may develop into a fascination with art and philosophical systems that better align with their expectations than the real world itself.

The third eye chakra is indigo blue in colour and Ayurveda recommends feeding it with blueberries, blackberries, grape juice and poppyseeds. Essential oils that benefit the third eye chakra include lavender, frankincense and bergamot. You can use these oils in a diffuser or dilute and apply them to the skin.

According to Indian teachings, the third eye chakra meditation should be performed with the eyes closed, with the breath directed to the space between the eyebrows to relax the third eye as profoundly as possible. Any meditation or form of everyday mindfulness is suitable for getting the third eye energy flowing, provided it fosters the connection between the thalamus' perceptive function and the energy regulation of the hypothalamus. Body-focused meditation and keeping a dream diary can help to strengthen inner perception and provide insight into the unconscious mind. Appropriate yoga poses include child's pose, eagle pose and thunderbolt pose.

The crown chakra (universal energy)

The crown chakra is the highest centre of energy, responsible for higher consciousness and connecting with universal energies. It is located above the top of the head, i.e., a little outside the body, within the energetic aura. It is often represented as a blooming lotus flower or a glowing crown. A balanced crown chakra can contribute to a deep understanding of existence, inner peace and spiritual growth.

Chapter fifteen of the *Bhagavad Gita* features a somewhat puzzling section about an 'inner tree'. It is described as immortal and those who scale it are believed to attain greater knowledge. In contrast to the tree that represents the gut and the navel chakra, this undying tree stands upside down. Its roots are located in our heads and look upwards because they are connected to the universe, while its trunk and branches reach down into the body, representing fleeting worries, troubles and desires. Scaling the tree means turning away from material aims and short-term goals and seeking higher things and universal values. In fact, the tree is a good stand-in for the crown chakra, uniting the nutritional energy from below with the spiritual energy from above. The crown chakra is associated with the pineal gland, which regulates circadian and other temporal rhythms via the messenger substances serotonin and melatonin, suggesting that the upside-down tree symbolises entry into a greater time and contact with the origin.

The crown chakra is purple; fittingly, dark cherries, which contain the sleep hormone melatonin, are also connected to this energy. According to Ayurveda, fragrances such as sandalwood, lotus, sage and juniper stimulate the crown chakra. In many spiritual traditions, fasting is a seasoned method for making contact with the inverted tree because it prompts us to explore nourishment that is not served on a plate. A headstand is a good option for advanced yogis who want to experience the brain as the root. The crown chakra meditation aims to explore our hidden inner self and multifaceted self and to experience our mysterious expansion into space. The visualisation for this chakra involves purple and white energies flowing down from above. This image ultimately enables us to understand why Hindu teaching does not view the chakral energies as a circulatory loop within the body, but as part of a more comprehensive current: transformations of nutritional energy are intended to integrate us into the circular flow of the cosmos.

Cleansing

The transformation of nutritional energies is never complete. There is always leftover food that cannot be converted and must be excreted. Removing this residue is crucial for our health because unprocessed residues can interact negatively with the body, leading to arterial and kidney calcification, arthrosis, or fatty liver.[1] We must also cleanse ourselves of specific higher energies, such as trapped heart energies, which may be expressed as alienation, desire, greed, hate and envy. There are similarities between certain practices for physical and mental cleansing; for instance, the use of heat in a sauna, which cleanses the body of excess micronutrients and negative feelings and tension. In this chapter, I aim to draw parallels between constipation and defecation and bodily hygiene and spiritual cleansing, including bowel cleanses, sweat lodges and tea ceremonies.

Let's briefly think back to how food is transformed inside our bodies: it undergoes four stages during which nutrients are broken down and new substances emerge. All these digestive processes are of utmost importance, as Claudia and Esther's tragic stories demonstrate. They were fed a diet of liquid food containing pure nutrients, circumventing these normal digestive processes and culminating in severe physical and psychological issues.

What is digestion? It begins in the mouth, where

we break down our food with our teeth and mix it with saliva, which contains digestive enzymes. Enzymes are proteins that our bodies produce to facilitate specific metabolic processes. The salivary enzyme amylase breaks down starch quickly, making it harder for bacteria that cause tooth decay to survive in the mouth. What's more, chewing, along with the taste and smell of foods, stimulates the stomach and gets the digestive juices flowing. The more mindfully we eat, the better this preparatory and cooperative process can work. Once our food arrives in our stomachs, it is broken down further and liquified by a combination of churning motions, stomach acid and other digestive enzymes. In the small intestine, bile acids from the liver and pancreatic juices help turn our food into a semi-liquid mush so the small intestine can convert and absorb the nutrients it contains. Next up is the large intestine, where bacteria help break down foods that are harder to digest. Our bodies produce around 75,000 enzymes, which control metabolic processes. By way of comparison, the bacteria in our gut have more than twenty million enzymes at their disposal. Thanks to them, digestion in the large intestine exhibits a degree of sophistication in breaking down, converting and producing new nutrients that we can hardly imagine. By contrast, eating isolated, simple nutrients, which are absorbed in the upper small intestine, means forgoing the much more powerful digestive machinery in the large intestine. Medically speaking, this is absolute madness, as it enables several pollutants to enter the body undigested – as in the cases of Claudia and Esther.

The course of digestion varies slightly depending on the nutrient. Digestion of carbohydrates begins in the mouth. However, the more complex the carbohydrate, the less capable the mouth is of breaking it down, meaning it must be processed more extensively and taken up further down in the gut. Some long-chain, complex carbohydrates can only be broken down by gut bacteria in the large intestine. These are known as prebiotics because they are required for gut flora to thrive. Digestion of fats can also begin in the mouth, aided by specific enzymes, but it mainly occurs in the small intestine with the help of bile acids from the liver and digestive juices from the pancreas. Proteins are broken down in the stomach by a specific enzyme and then processed in the small intestine. The size of the macronutrients and the grid-like system that holds them together, the food matrix, has a significant part to play here; it is these that decide how and where nutrients are broken down and what substances they are transformed into. Whole foods have the advantage of reaching the large intestine, where they are refined and transformed in a much more complex way than they would be in the mouth, stomach, or small intestine.

At the end of the process comes defecation, the excretion of waste from the digestive tract via the anus. This complex exercise requires the gastrointestinal tract, the enteric nervous system, the sacral plexus and the muscles of the abdomen, back, pelvis, respiratory system and legs to all work together. The process begins with the stool being transported from the large intestine to the rectum, triggering the defecation reflex: the rectum contracts and the anus relaxes. Defecation occurs without the need for conscious control, with a movement from the large intestine to the inner part of the anus, where smooth muscles push the stool outwards. However, once the stool reaches the outer part of the anus, defecation becomes a consciously controlled process, making it possible for us to withhold our stool if necessary. Defecation is a fascinating instance of cooperation between conscious and unconscious processes and it is here where mindfulness offers us the opportunity to coordinate these processes in the best possible way.

Mindful defecation

I have developed a toilet meditation that aims to make defecation easier, in the hope of supporting people suffering from constipation, IBS and other gastro-intestinal issues. I use the acronym *FIRST* to remember the steps. It is also advisable to put your feet up on a toilet stool to ensure your knees are higher than your hips. This relaxes the bowel muscles and helps to empty the bowel fully.

- F stands for feelings. This first step is about becoming conscious of your thoughts, feelings and bodily sensations. It's best to start at the bottom and slowly work your way up: *how are my feet feeling? How does it feel in the gaps between my toes? How do my shins, knees, thighs, pelvis, abdomen and lower back feel? Where exactly is my body making contact with the toilet seat?* When urinating, whether seated or standing, it is essential to return to your feet and focus on the contact they make with your shoes and the ground. *What feelings does it bring up to move through my body in this way? What thoughts am I having? How deeply am I breathing?*

• I stands for imagine. For this step, it helps to visualise your pelvis, rectum, stool and anus. You might also imagine the stool as a living being that is trying to find its way out of your body. When urinating, you can visualise your bladder and the liquid inside it, which is trying to flow back into the Earth's water cycle. Imagine your bowel and bladder as complete, powerful and capable – ready to work together.

• R stands for relaxation. Defecation depends on relaxing the whole body, particularly the pelvic floor and anus. It's good to check in with your body, working from top to bottom: *how loose are my face and jaw muscles? Are the muscles of my neck and shoulders relaxed? How do my hands and fingers feel? Are my abdomen, my legs and my feet relaxed?* As you do this, you should feel your breath in your stomach. One long exhalation will help relax both the body and the mind. If you are having trouble relaxing, running the tap can help, as the sound of flowing water is soothing and helps the mind anticipate a bowel movement.

• S stands for surrender. It's crucial to consciously allow and enable the bowel and the bladder to empty. As described above, we can deliberately stop the defecation process. Tackling this resistance enables the organs to perform their natural cleansing function. Surrendering also means becoming soft, both mentally and physically. And often, that's all it takes. Sometimes, however, conscious pressure, a change of position, or deep breathing can be helpful too. You might try a certain degree of pushing down, but proceeding mindfully and gently should be at the forefront, taking an approach based on respectful cooperation rather than force. Mindful observation of the body can help support a gentle approach.

• T stands for thankfulness. Like any successful cooperative process, we should feel thankful for our partner at the end – our partner, in this case, being our body, specifically our bowel. It is an opportunity to be proud of having carried out a natural process efficiently and successfully. The body will demonstrate its gratitude with a feeling of relief and, sometimes, even joy. The reasons behind these reactions are both mechanical and neurological. Defecation relieves internal pressure on the lower abdomen, allowing the muscles of the gut, bladder and pelvic floor to relax. It also stimulates the vagus nerve, which runs from the brain stem to the large intestine. Activating the vagus nerve can provoke light shaking, create a sensation of warmth and even lower blood pressure. On a neurological level, stimulating the vagus nerve has a soothing and anxiety-relieving effect on the brain. All these factors contribute to an increased sense of well-being, which predominantly manifests following an extensive bowel movement. It explains why passing a bowel movement is often a satisfying and pleasant experience.

Having defecated, it's worth taking a good look at what you have just produced. A healthy stool is typically firm, smooth and sausage-like in shape, but soft enough to pass effortlessly without intense pressure on the bowel. Delaying going to the toilet can cause the body to extract water from the stool, making it more difficult to pass. It is therefore important to develop a degree of bowel mindfulness throughout the day to avoid missing the natural defecation reflex. If the reflex is not particularly pronounced, it can help to drink a glass of water or tea before breakfast.

A hard stool, combined with straining, can cause health problems such as chronic constipation, haemorrhoids and anal fissures. An adult's stool should usually be brown. Bright red in the stool may indicate fresh blood from the lower digestive tract or anus. Black stools can be caused by eating certain foods, such as blueberries, liquorice, or iron tablets, but can also be a sign of bleeding in the upper digestive tract, with the blood turning dark during digestion. If you experience sudden changes in your stool or pain while defecating that occur for no apparent reason and do not improve within a few days, contact your doctor.

To what extent does nutritional and environmental waste contaminate our bodies?

We are currently witnessing a boom in detox treatments, which assume that our bodies struggle to expel food residue and require extra help in the form of teas, fruit juices, enemas, intestinal cleansing, or laxatives. When I was studying medicine, I wanted to get a clearer picture of how waste works in the human body, so I carefully examined the cadavers we were dissecting for impurities. Still, I couldn't find any evidence of harmful buildup. In fact, if defecation is working normally, our bowels can thoroughly cleanse themselves of food residues. Instead, many cadavers I observed had large quantities of fatty tissue, filling large parts of the abdomen and surrounding the stomach, liver and intestines. This is also known as belly fat or visceral fat and, according to studies, raises the risk of heart conditions and Type 2 diabetes more than subcutaneous fat. Visceral fat can also surround the heart, limiting its flexibility. This confirms once again how important it is not to eat too much and to prevent a build-up of stomach fat with a regular, healthy and mindful diet, as laid out in the previous chapters.

Using a microscope during my investigations, I noticed that not only had the fat cells surrounded the organs, but they had also migrated into the organs, penetrating them. This is particularly striking in cases of fatty liver, where every single liver cell contains droplets of fat. This makes the liver heavy and taut, reducing its detoxification capacity. The leading cause of fatty liver is a sustained diet high in sugar and other short-chain carbohydrates. Excessive alcohol consumption (more than a glass of wine a day for women and two glasses for men) may also increase the risk of alcoholic fatty liver disease. Alcohol is a liver toxin and very high in calories. This combination quickly leads to fat permeating the liver and impairs its proper function. This has serious consequences as the liver is the body's primary detoxifying organ: if a person's liver fails, they will die within hours. The liver converts pollutants that evade gut bacteria into harmless substances and also disposes of excess blood cells. Over time, accumulated fats can cause inflammation and damage to the liver because the liver interprets these fats as foreign bodies, leading to cirrhosis, in which liver cells are replaced by scar tissue. All these processes, which are caused by liver fat, raise the risk of liver cancer. However, fatty liver is not caused by the food we eat, which immediately pollutes and clogs up our bodies. It is a vicious cycle: eating unhealthy foods and eating too much, along with drinking alcohol, inhibits the body's natural detoxifying processes, which makes an unhealthy life-style even more harmful to our bodies, which, in turn, are rendered more vulnerable.

Alongside an increase in fat deposits, another issue I noticed in my painstaking examinations of cadavers was a hardening of the larger blood vessels, such as the aorta and the leg arteries. It was a strikingly tactile experience to observe the thickening of the vessel walls, almost as hard as bone and the stiffness of these otherwise elastic tubes. It immediately became clear to me why hardened blood vessels are the most common cause of death. It is a significant challenge for the heart to circulate blood through a system of stiffened channels. It only takes a few minor changes for a stiff and narrow channel of this kind to collapse or narrow, interrupting blood flow. We particularly fear this kind of calcification of the blood vessels when it occurs in the heart, in the coronary arteries. A blockage here causes parts of the heart muscle to die instantly. Under the microscope, the arterial walls will exhibit many fibres containing fat stores, leading them to be often inflamed and calcified. This is known as arteriosclerosis and begins with fatty deposits in the arterial walls that restrict blood flow. A vicious cycle emerges: the more fat that is stored, the higher a person's blood pressure rises, which in turn leads to more damage and more fat deposits. The main causes of this are smoking, obesity and inadequate physical activity. As I have mentioned many times before, the body does not like having full stores or excess tissue. When these are present, the body increasingly views fat deposits as foreign bodies, leading to inflammation. Unlike the liver, however, it is not just fascia or connective tissue that is stored in fat; calcium deposits are stored there too. A second vicious circle begins: the greater the calcification, the harder the arteries become, prompting a further rise in blood pressure, which in turn encourages further calcification.

Medicine has developed several treatments to halt this process, including antihypertensives and medications (statins) which prevent and partly reverse fat build-up in the arteries, as well as surgical methods for removing hardening and calcification, for instance in the carotid artery. There are also indications that a diet of whole fruits and vegetables may prevent fat build-up and calcification of blood vessels and even reverse them.[2]

This is due to the antioxidant and anti-inflammatory compounds in food, which help counter inflammation in arterial walls. According to preliminary findings, the thousands of purifying substances in tomatoes may be particularly effective in preventing arterial calcification. This might be why people in the Mediterranean Blue Zones, where tomatoes are eaten at almost every meal, exhibit a relatively low incidence of heart attacks.

I didn't find any accumulated plastics in the cadavers I examined – except for surgical sutures – but our increasing consumption of microplastics presents another challenge for our bodies. Mussels filter the food they eat out of seawater in coastal areas and consequently contain large amounts of plastic. In Europe, Belgians eat the most molluscs per capita, with moules frites among their national dishes. As a result, Belgians consume, on average, 11,000 microplastic particles per annum. We still know very little about the possible harm this may cause. The plastic does not appear to accumulate in the gut, but it is sure to have a negative impact on gut flora. Research on animals fed microplastics has shown that this can lead to problems with the gut-blood barrier, decreased bacterial diversity, increased numbers of unusual, plastic-loving bacteria and inflammatory responses.[3]

Unlike the gut, the lungs are much less capable of expelling waste. In Western industrialised nations, we breathe in the equivalent of a credit card's worth of microplastics every year. This plastic does not simply disappear; it can be observed in autopsies and during operations, embedded in deep areas of the lungs. Rust and tobacco particles also accumulate in the lungs. Waste products of this kind all cause inflammation, which impairs breathing and raises the risk of lung cancer in the long term.[4] It is one of the reasons why smoking is so unhealthy, reducing life expectancy by around ten years. To maintain and promote our body's natural processes of self-cleaning, it is worth taking regular walks in nature, through gardens, fields and forests, where the air is naturally purified, particularly after rainfall. When we breathe, we must do so not just with our chests, as this can lead to chest muscle cramping and less air reaching the lower parts of the lungs. Abdominal breathing is a better approach, as it helps to cleanse the pulmonary lobes and activates the vagus nerve, promoting the production of cleansing mucus inside the lungs and inhibiting inflammation. Exercise, saunas and breathing exercises can also help to improve breathing. One good practice is to take a brief pause after breathing in, before breathing out slowly. It can help to count while you do this: count to four as you breathe in, pause for four more, then count to eight as you breathe out. It is also crucial to regularly air out your living room, bedroom and workspace to ensure you are breathing in as much oxygen as possible and as little dust and toxins as possible.

What should we make of enemas and bowel cleanses?

Due to the possible presence of pollutants in our food and a lack of confidence in the body's natural processes for cleansing the bowel, an increasing number of people have come to view occasional enemas or cleanses as a sensible option for managing their health. In conventional medicine, enemas are often used to prepare the bowel for medical examinations, such as a colonoscopy. However, some alternative practitioners recommend enemas for other purposes, such as detoxifying the body. It is important to emphasise, however, that enemas or bowel cleanses are carried out only very rarely on grounds of medical necessity. As I have described above, waste does not accumulate in the gut and, providing our gut flora is intact and contains a variety of enzymes, it does an exceptionally efficient job of processing and excreting harmful substances. Colonic irrigation often involves flushing large volumes of water enriched with herbs, coffee, or other additives through the gut. This is performed using a tube introduced into the rectum. In some cases, small amounts of water remain in the large intestine for a short time before being removed. Adherents of bowel cleansing practices claim that deposits in the gastro-intestinal tract may cause various health problems, such as arthritis and high blood pressure. They believe that bowel cleanses improve overall health by removing these deposits, boosting energy and fortifying the immune system. Yet there is no scientific evidence for deposits of this kind. In healthy people, the body's natural process of defecation, in collaboration with the gut flora, seems to be highly effective until well into old age. In fact, bowel cleanses may even be harmful, as the gut lining is very large, thin and sensitive and cleansing solutions could disturb the mucous membrane, gut bacteria and the body's natural fluid balance. There have also been cases reported of people dying after undergoing coffee enemas because coffee contains substances such as caffeine and acids, which can irritate the gut membrane, leaving it overstimulated and inflamed. This may cause bleeding, ulcers, or even holes in the gut wall. Side effects can also include cramps, gas, diarrhoea, nausea and vomiting. Bowel cleanses should therefore only be carried out under a doctor's supervision and with full consideration of the possible risks.

The mysterious sensation of constipation

Now that I have hopefully allayed any fears about clogged bowels and dampened any sense of optimism about the curative potential of enemas, I'd like to turn my attention to a widespread complaint: constipation. Many people suffer from chronic constipation. Despite this problem being so widespread, there is no coherent definition for the condition itself. Some doctors look to the frequency of bowel movements: typically, a patient reporting fewer than three bowel movements per week will be diagnosed with constipation. The problem with this definition, however, is that we usually severely underestimate the frequency of our bowel movements because we are not mindful of our toilet habits and tend instead to distract ourselves. This is precisely the kind of situation where keeping a stool diary and having a regular *FIRST* meditation practice could help to provide a reliable idea of stool frequency. The second problem with the above definition is that the frequency of one's stools merely indicates the speed of bowel function and it may just as easily point to a bowel disorder or paralysis. Nine out of ten people complaining of constipation report a normal transit time, meaning the time it takes for food to be excreted after eating. The average transit time is 2.4 days for women and 1.9 days for men, distributed as follows: one to three hours in the stomach, two to six hours in the small intestine and one to three days in the large intestine. The large intestine is granted the greatest amount of time for digestion – another indicator of the importance of a diet of whole foods, since the large intestine boasts the most enzymes, for optimal digestion. Industrially processed foods bypass this essential process of transformation and purification in the large intestine because they lack a food matrix and are absorbed by the small intestine within a matter of hours. Paradoxically, this extends transit times because nothing reaches the large intestine, so whatever is stored there remains there longer.

Some rare bowel conditions exhibit significantly prolonged transit times, such as Hirschsprung's disease, a serious developmental condition of the enteric nervous system characterised by severe swelling of the stomach and a lack of bowel movements from birth. Prolonged transit times are also typical in cases of women with constipation who only experience occasional bowel movements (once a week or less). The problem often begins in puberty. A fibre-rich diet can help increase stool weight and reduce large intestinal transit time, alleviating constipation. However, people experiencing significantly prolonged transit times due to a bowel condition respond poorly to dietary fibre. In cases such as these, a visit to the doctor is advisable.

If you find yourself suffering from persistent constipation, it can be worth getting to know your own transit time. Unfortunately, obtaining a precise measurement of your transit time is fairly laborious: patients swallow small, radiopaque markers at regular intervals and undergo repeated X-rays of the stomach to get an accurate estimate of the gut's transport speed.

However, there is a much simpler, if less precise, method of doing this and it can be done at home. All you have to do is eat two muffins, both dyed with royal blue food colouring. You then wait to see how long it takes before you pass a blue stool. Transit times for healthy people can vary from half a day to four days. The same studies also show that people with longer transit times tend to have more belly fat and exhibit large spikes in blood sugar and fat after eating, which can contribute significantly to arterial calcification. It underlines the importance of daily physical activity – a thirty-minute walk is a good start – and of eating whole foods with plenty of fibre to ensure your transit time is not unnecessarily prolonged.[5]

Many who suffer from constipation do not view their condition in terms of the lack of frequency of their bowel movements but in terms of problems they experience when they do go to the toilet, such as having to strain, hard, lumpy stools, a feeling of not having properly voided their bowels, bloating and a swollen stomach. Since most cases of constipation present with normal bowel frequency and transit time, medicine is increasingly defining constipation based on these symptoms. It is imperative to monitor stool consistency. As I have said, a healthy stool should look like a smooth sausage with a rough exterior. Hard lumps suggest constipation, while soft lumps and small scraps of stool point to diarrhoea. An occasional, passing episode of constipation is very typical, however. Problems only arise once it becomes chronic, because a hard stool can injure the anus, leading to pain and anxiety about going to the toilet, which only makes the constipation worse.

Since a diet of whole, fibre-rich foods (such as sweetcorn, plums and kiwi), increased water intake and physical activity are key ways to soften one's stool, the question occasionally arises as to whether seeing corn kernels in the toilet bowl indicates a problem. Fortunately, this is not the case; if anything, it's a sign of a healthy diet. Finding undigested food particles in your stool indicates that the large intestine is adequately nourished and challenged by the food you eat, which serves as a stimulus to improve its function. Only a marked increase in undigested food in your stool suggests a possible digestive complaint, such as diarrhoea, inflammation of the bowel, or irritable bowel.

Not every case of constipation is related to diet. Around a fifth of people who suffer from chronic constipation struggle with a bowel voidance disorder that cannot be traced back exclusively to diet. This kind of constipation is often caused by anal fissures, haemorrhoids, a lack of coordination or weakness in the pelvic floor muscles or cramping in the pelvic floor. Factors such as exaggerated hygiene practices, pregnancy and sexual abuse also have a part to play. Long-standing injuries around the anus should be assessed and treated by a doctor. Pilates, pelvic floor therapy and biofeedback therapy have proven to be effective in treating disorders of the pelvic floor muscles. Sitz baths, particularly cold-water baths and hot-and-cold contrast baths, are another effective way to treat sluggishness in the pelvic area and to increase awareness of bowel movements. As I mentioned at the beginning of this chapter, preventing defecation disorders requires a fibre-rich diet and a mindful and conscious approach to bowel movements. This method entails a kind of natural biofeedback, meaning that potential complaints can be recognised early and optimal relaxation can prevent injuries in the area around the anus.

Laxatives are the most common medicinal treatment for constipation and are used to support excretion. They work in several different ways. Bulking agents such as psyllium, linseed and wheat are used to make the stool larger and softer, but they can also cause flatulence and bloating, particularly at the beginning of treatment. It is also important for sufferers to drink plenty of water to prevent hard stools, which can worsen constipation. Laxative salt mixtures, such as Glauber's salt and Epsom salts, increase the amount of water in the gut, making the stool softer and more lubricated. Diarrhoea is the most common side-effect of this treatment. In older people, excessive salt intake may disrupt the body's salt balance. Then some laxatives directly stimulate the bowel, causing it to move more and produce more mucous. The disadvantage of these is that, over time, the bowel becomes accustomed to the treatment and can weaken, even becoming more listless. Overall, a fibre-rich diet of whole foods remains a preferable option.

The whole body plays a part in the cleansing process.

Like the gut, the skin is another important excretory organ, so it is worth caring for your skin and cleaning it regularly to remove dead skin cells and waste products that build up when we sweat. Next up are the kidneys – so important to our body's internal cleanliness that we have two of them. The kidneys filter waste and harmful substances from the blood, maintain the balance of water and salt, excrete excess acids and bases and regulate blood pressure. A person can lose all function in one kidney and still survive because the other kidney, assuming it is working well, can do the job alone. The best way to support your kidneys is to drink plenty of clean water.

Under normal conditions (diet, exercise and climate), a healthy person will produce at least half a litre of urine per day. Fluid intake of more than half a litre will lead to a person excreting pure water. The notion that we are all profoundly dehydrated – and the recommendation that we drink as much as possible – does not have a basis in scientific study. In fact, the opposite can be true: filtering excessive amounts of water from the blood puts strain on the kidneys and may lead to wear and tear over the years. For most young and healthy people, the best approach is to drink when you feel thirsty. Our feelings of thirst naturally increase in hot weather or when we exercise. However, older people must ensure they drink plenty, as a person's sense of thirst can decrease after the age of seventy.

The lymphatic system is another important cleansing mechanism in the body, transporting interstitial fluid from tissues back into the bloodstream. The liquid flows through the lymph nodes, where it is tested for pathogens and cleaned. The lymphatic system also absorbs nutrients – particularly fats – in the intestinal tract and makes them available to the body. Unlike blood, lymph does not have a pump transporting it through vessels that reach into every corner of the body. Instead, the flow of lymph is powered by the surrounding muscles and the movement of the breath. This is why physical activity and mindful breathing help cleanse the body.

Are periods cleansing?

When my daughter reached puberty, she showed me a pad with red blood on it. 'But what's this for?' she asked. On the spur of the moment, I replied, 'It's a kind of cleaning'. It was only later that I realised that this was only part of a more extensive answer. Doctors in antiquity, such as Galen of Pergamon, claimed that what women excreted each month was 'excess' blood. In fact, iron excretion could be one reason why women live longer than men, if we are going by the rule of thumb that empty stores are better in the long term than full ones, which applies primarily to iron. The disadvantage is that periods can cause anaemia, which may sometimes require treatment with iron, particularly if it leads to tiredness and exhaustion. The second kind of cleansing that occurs here is of bacteria that may be introduced to the womb by sperm following sexual intercourse, which is then flushed out during menstruation.

But while it may serve to cleanse blood and bacteria, one question remains: why is menstruation so rare in nature? Most mammals, except for a few species of apes and bats, do not menstruate. New research offers clues as to why, suggesting that, in humans, the mother and foetus live in very close proximity for an extended period, sharing several blood vessels and immune cells. The mother's mucous membrane is only able to be so open to her child if it is destroyed and regrown every month in preparation for a possible pregnancy.[6]

Period blood is particularly interesting because it contains proteins that promote tissue repair. At present, attempts are being made to use these proteins to treat wound healing disorders, such as after burns or operations. Hildegard von Bingen, whose concept of greening power we encountered earlier in the book, seemed to understand all of this intuitively, writing: 'For woman, the rivulet of menstruation indicates her greenness and flowering that blooms in her offspring. As a tree from its greenness brings forth blossoms and leaves and bears fruit, so too woman, from the greenness of the rivulets of menstrual blood, brings forth blossoms and leaves in the fruit of her womb …'[7] Hildegard was the first to recognise that the processes of excretion and blossoming belonged together and she also dared to hold fast to this idea and teach it to others.

A mindful approach to bodily odours

A mindful appreciation of bodily odours can help us to recognise complaints and illnesses early. A sweet-smelling breath can point to a bacterial infection. A sweet, putrid scent, for example, is associated with scarlet fever, a disease that presents with a sore throat, fever and a bumpy 'strawberry tongue', and responds well to antibiotics. Breath that smells like fresh bread is a sign of typhoid, an infection caused by the bacterium Salmonella typhi, which is usually transmitted through dirty water and characterised by diarrhoea, constipation and skin changes. Left untreated, typhoid can lead to severe complications, including intestinal perforation and sepsis, making early diagnosis and treatment with antibiotics all the more vital.

Sour-smelling breath can point to reflux disease, where stomach acid flows up into the oesophagus. A simple way to combat this is to raise the head of the bed, so stomach acid stays in the stomach overnight. Breath that smells of fruit and acetone indicates a metabolic disorder characterised by swift fat burning, typically caused by a lack of insulin due to diabetes, or a lack of carbohydrates, in the case of extreme ketogenic diets. The acetone scent comes from ketones, which are healthy in small amounts and do not usually affect the breath. Treatment typically involves administering fluids and insulin.

Breath that smells like ammonia can point to kidney disease, in which the kidneys do not excrete waste products, leading them to accumulate in the blood before being exhaled. Breath that smells like raw liver, clay, or rotten eggs can indicate acute liver disease. If any of these odours persist, it is advisable to visit a doctor, who can check liver and kidney function with a simple blood test.

An animal-like smell on the skin, often accompanied by notes of musk, is a very early sign of Parkinson's disease and can occur long before any motor disorder becomes visible. The smell is caused by changes in sebum production on the upper back and forehead. If you suspect this, it is worth seeking help from your GP or a neurologist. A fishy scent from the penis or vagina points to dysbiosis, an imbalance of the gut flora. Sex organs ought to be slightly acidic to protect them against harmful bacteria and a fishy scent suggests that this protective acid is absent. Washing and changing your underwear regularly can help remedy the problem.

Rather than being a sign of a serious illness, bad breath is more frequently caused by an imbalance of flora in the mouth. Unfortunately, people become accustomed to the smell and often don't notice it themselves. To check whether you have bad breath, it's worth asking someone close to you or carrying out a test yourself. To do this, lick your wrist or the back of your hand, then wait ten seconds before smelling the area of skin that has just dried.

Our mouths contain vast numbers of bacteria – considerably more than the anus, because the insides of our mouths provide the perfect environment for them: dark, warm and moist. The food and drink we consume also provides these bacteria with a plentiful supply of nutrients. Industrially processed foods may contain high quantities of sugar, enabling harmful bacteria to multiply and suppress other healthy, protective bacteria. These harmful bacteria love our teeth and gums, colonising them intensively and increasing the risk of tooth cavities and gum inflammation. Yet the harmful bacteria in our mouths can have a negative impact on our entire bodies, raising the risk of fatigue, Type 2 diabetes, heart conditions, respiratory infections and disorders of the brain. In theory, this makes kissing downright dangerous, due to the risk of encountering unfriendly bacteria. However, you're much more likely to experience the positive effects of kissing, as the practice itself increases the diversity of mouth bacteria.

Caring mindfully for our bodies, from head to toe

Sugar is the leading cause of unhappy mouth flora, so it is worth brushing your teeth after every meal or snack. It's mostly a case of mechanically removing sticky sugars and the unhealthy bacteria that cling to our teeth.

Many toothpastes contain fluoride, which naturally protects teeth against acid-forming bacteria. Gently massaging the gums can also promote circulation and prevent gingival atrophy. But cleaning your teeth after every meal isn't the only thing you can do to benefit your teeth – microfasting until your next meal is a good practice, too. After all, you don't want to have to spend the whole day brushing your teeth.

The nasopharynx forms the upper part of the respiratory tract. Like the mouth, it is a body part that has direct contact with the outside world, meaning it is regularly exposed to harmful bacteria and viruses. Nasal irrigation is considered one of the most effective ways to protect yourself against colds and allergies and it also improves the sense of smell, which, as we know, plays a vital role in mindful eating. It's easy to make up a cleansing solution yourself: mix a teaspoon of table salt with distilled or boiled and cooled water (or good tap water). To rinse out your nose, turn your head to one side over the sink and place the nasal irrigation spout in your upper nostril. Breathing through your mouth, carefully pour the saltwater solution into your upper nostril, letting it flow out of the lower nostril. You can then repeat the process from the other side. This technique was familiar to ancient Ayurvedic sages, who developed the neti pot for this purpose. You can find neti pots in pharmacies, health food shops and online. Saltwater nasal sprays work similarly by moistening the nose, but they do not have the same cleansing effect as nasal irrigation. If the nose is very dry, Ayurveda recommends treating this with sesame oil – a treatment for nasal dryness also favoured by conventional medicine.

Our feet are two parts of our bodies that are in direct contact with our environment. As such, it is sensible to wash your feet before bed, especially if you do not have time for a shower or bath. All you need is some warm water, a washcloth and soap. I use shea butter soap, but if you have rough heels or calluses, you might benefit from a soap containing pumice. The washing of feet is widespread in many spiritual traditions and serves to strengthen both body and mind. Aside from that, it's lovely to wash your feet at the end of a long day; it's refreshing, cooling and a good way to prevent impurities from entering your body through your soles. It is also an excellent opportunity for a bit of mindfulness before going to bed. Take your time and concentrate on the gaps between your toes, the soles of your feet, your toe knuckles and your insteps before thoroughly drying your feet.

The purifying effects of sleep

In 2004, I was a young researcher working in the US. When I managed to show an association between sleeping less than six hours per night and consistent weight gain, my findings were met with an enormous media response.[8] Numerous journalists called to talk to me about my 'revolutionary' discovery. And yet, a team of Spanish scientists had documented the negative effects of insufficient sleep on the body's metabolism just a few years earlier. Still, the media had overlooked it, perhaps because our study of young adults was of greater interest to their audience. Since then, hundreds of studies have been published on this phenomenon and we are now much better informed as to the cleansing function that sleep performs.

I have already discussed the importance of the lymphatic system, but recent findings suggest that a similar system exists in the brain as well. This is known as the glymphatic system because it works a little differently. The brain does not contain any muscles that might regulate lymph flow; instead, brain cells contract slightly during sleep, causing the spaces between them to grow. This allows waste products, toxins and excess micronutrients such as calcium, zinc and selenium to be filtered from the brain more efficiently. It is why bed rest helps reduce the risk of diseases of the brain.[9]

Yet sleep has another vital role to play: it allows the brain to delete unnecessary memories and better organise important experiences, storing them as engrams. This process is essential for survival and involves reactivating old memories to give the brain a second opportunity to reassess their emotional significance and determine if they are burdensome or gratifying. The time we spend sleeping is limited, so the brain has developed a memory player of sorts, which plays back memories five to twenty times faster. Dreams can offer insights into this cleansing process.[10]

Sleep isn't just of central importance to the brain; it is essential to the recovery of the whole body. Many hormones follow a daily rhythm. Levels of the stress hormone, for instance, drop at night and increase in the morning to prepare us for the day ahead. In addition, the body releases more melatonin and certain growth hormones at night, promoting growth, cell repair and tissue renewal. Sleep also gives the liver the time and energy it needs to process the toxins and waste products that have accumulated throughout the day.

The latest findings also indicate that less sleep and irregular sleep can disrupt gut bacteria, increasing the risk of weight gain and metabolic disorders. A lack of sleep also weakens the gut-blood barrier, increasing the risk of inflammatory processes and autoimmune diseases. Intact gut flora offers protection against neurotoxins such as lead, cadmium and mercury. Consequently, sleep problems can make people more sensitive to these harmful substances.[11]

However, people who have trouble falling asleep or who frequently wake up in the night should not be too concerned about these processes of cleansing and renewal. What matters most is the rest and inactivity that comes with lying down and it's important to go to bed at the same time every night and get up at the same time in the morning. Studies also show that earlier bedtimes are associated with a reduced tendency to consume unnecessary calories.

Spiritual cleansing in a sweat lodge

Much like sleep, primitive spiritual and shamanistic methods of cleansing go hand in hand with the experience of altered consciousness. One enduring example of this tradition is the centuries-old ritual of sweat lodges, practised by First Nations peoples of North and Central America. The practice involves a small, beehive-shaped hut, often made from willow branches, sticks and animal furs or blankets, typically erected by a group in an open space. Building the hut together fosters a sense of togetherness and reconciliation in the community.

The sweat lodge itself may be small, but according to shamanistic belief, it holds up a mirror to the entire universe, where human beings merge with the spirit world. The person in charge of the fire will place stones in the pit in the middle of the hut, which have been heated in a fire outside. The choice of stones and the heat they give off is crucial if the ritual is to be a success. The master of ceremonies pours water over the hot stones to create steam, then burns aromatic herbs to enhance the purifying effects of the steam. In a way, it resembles the process of cooking: time, heat, moisture and herbs determine what happens to the raw, unfinished 'ingredients' inside. The sweat that follows is seen as a process of detoxification and renewal. Participants perform prayers and chants to call on helpful spirits to support their purification. The smells and the heat can help dissolve any sense of self-preoccupation and enable participants to experience a spiritual feeling of being elevated as part of a larger whole. Tahca Ushte, a Sioux medicine man, describes the experience as follows: 'There is a great surge of power. You inhale that breath, drink in the water, the white steam. It represents clouds, the living soul, life.'[12] The ritual ends with the participants leaving the hut like newborns, symbolically cleansed and renewed in the womb of the great Mother, as the sweat lodge represents it through seclusion, darkness and warmth.

The Japanese tea ceremony

In Japan, the tea ceremony is a deeply-rooted cultural practice that is about much more than simply drinking tea. Like the sweat lodge, it has a spiritual, cleansing element intended to maintain and foster respect and harmony among its participants. Every aspect of the ceremony is aesthetically and spiritually significant: the choice of utensils, the arrangement of the space and the way the tea is served. The ceremony follows a strict sequence, from the way the tea is prepared to the moment it is drunk and every step is carried out with utmost care and attentiveness, emphasising the beauty in simplicity and everyday life.

Before entering the teahouse, participants wash their hands and rinse their mouths to free themselves from 'the dust of the everyday'. During the ceremony, the tea master slowly and carefully cleans the utensils in the presence of the guests, indicating that the process is about cleansing in a higher sense. Finally, after several other steps, each guest receives a tea bowl, which they hold with both hands, turning it around and drinking the tea slowly and mindfully in a few sips.

The famous master of the Japanese tea ceremony, Okakura Tenshin, described his experience of being a guest at a tea ceremony in striking terms: 'The first cup moistens my lips and throat, the second cup breaks my loneliness, the third cup searches my barren entrail but to find therein some 5,000 volumes of odd ideographs. The fourth cup raises a slight perspiration – all the wrong of life passes away through my pores. At the fifth cup, I am purified; the sixth cup calls me to the realms of the immortals.'[13] This brief quote alone demonstrates that, in a tea ceremony, the cleansing of lips and mouth coincides with the higher cleansing of the soul, expanding consciousness in a cosmic manner.

The tea ceremony ritual can be traced back to Buddhism, which places great importance on the act of cleansing oneself of negative karma. This is founded on the notion that evil deeds and negative emotions give rise to further bad actions and feelings. Parallels can be found in neuroscientific studies showing that patterns of behaviour can be developed and reinforced, which, for instance, form the neuronal foundation for addictive behaviours. The Buddhist practice offers various methods for cleansing oneself of bad karma, including mindful eating, consciously exploring hunger and thirst, making targeted changes to negative behaviours and practising serenity in unpleasant situations. Requests for forgiveness can also aid inner cleansing. Similarly, in Christianity, openly confessing to transgressions against others is a well-known method of catharsis. Reconciliation is an integral way to cleanse oneself of the bitterness and resentment that alienate us from the flow of life.

Conclusion

In today's world, food is often reduced to numbers – calories, grams, macros. But what truly nourishes us is more complex and more intelligent than any isolated nutrient. Throughout this book, we've explored the idea that health arises not from individual substances, but from the interaction of nutrients within the structure of real food – the food matrix – and how this interacts with the wisdom of the human body.

A whole nut nourishes differently than the same nutrients in a pill. A fermented cheese, a traditional grain, or a wild vegetable carries layers of complexity – physical, microbial and cultural – that no ultra-processed imitation can reproduce. Our bodies have evolved over millennia in dialogue with such complexity. It is not just the what, but the how of food that matters: its texture, structure, preparation and the context in which we eat.

This is why nutrient diversity is not a luxury, but a biological necessity. The more varied, unrefined and close to nature our foods are, the more they support the gut's microbial ecosystem, regulate immune function and engage the deep intelligence of the body. Our digestive system is not a passive tube – it is an active sensory organ, constantly interpreting what we ingest in terms of safety, energy, rhythm and memory.

To eat well, then, is not only to choose 'healthy' ingredients, but to engage with food as a living system. It means reconnecting to natural structures – fibres, textures, bonds – that the industrial food system tends to dismantle. It also means valuing diversity: not just in nutrients, but in tastes, colours and even in emotional tone.

True nourishment happens when food supports our inner regulation – when it feeds not just the body, but the gut-brain connection, the immune balance and our sense of rhythm and well-being. And this doesn't require perfection. It requires presence, variety and a reconnection to real food – food your grandmother would recognise, as Michael Pollan put it, but also food your gut bacteria would recognise as familiar, meaningful and alive.

This book invites a shift: away from control and correction and toward curiosity and complexity. Toward food that is not only functional, but packed full of life, full of diversity, full of meaning.

To return to what nourishes us is to return to food as relationship – and to the deep, embodied intelligence that connects us with ourselves, with nature and with others.

GLOSSARY

Blue Zones

Blue Zones are regions of the world where people live longer, on average, and enjoy a higher quality of life. These places are typically characterised by specific foods, cooking traditions, eating habits, social cohesion and the temporal sequences of life (regular patterns of sleeping and waking and regular mealtimes). Examples of Blue Zone regions include Sardinia (Italy), Okinawa (Japan), the Nicoya Peninsula (Costa Rica) and Icaria (Greece). Research into these areas can provide insights into the factors that contribute to a long and healthy life.

The gut-brain connection

The gut-brain connection, or gut-brain axis, is a complex communication system that exists between the gastrointestinal tract and the central nervous system, with information flowing in both directions. The gut acts as a sensory organ, supplying data to the brain and simultaneously receiving signals from the brain to control digestion. The autonomic nervous system, particularly the vagus nerve and the sympathetic nervous system, provides the axis's fast connections. The gut uses hormones to furnish the brain with information about food quality, digestibility, hunger and satiety. A significant part of the immune system is also located in the gut, where it uses chemical signals (cytokines) to send information about potential pathogens to the brain. Gut bacteria can produce substances, such as butyric acid, that directly affect brain function. New research suggests that the gut-brain connection plays a role in regulating mood, sleep and even cognitive processes. Additionally, there is increasing evidence that disruptions to the gut-brain connection may underlie certain brain diseases.

The gluten framework

Gluten is the name given to the proteins present in certain kinds of grains, particularly wheat, barley and rye. When flour is mixed with water, these proteins form a viscous network or chemical framework. This network gives dough its elastic structure, retaining the gas produced during proofing and contributing to the delicate structure and shape of bread and other baked goods. The gluten framework binds nutrients together, slowing their digestion and absorption, which is beneficial for our health. Durum wheat products and sourdough bread both boast particularly good gluten frameworks, making them healthier overall. People with coeliac disease are obliged to avoid foods containing gluten. In contrast, people with gluten intolerance should avoid gluten-free products, as these have no gluten framework, making them less healthy.

The food matrix

The food matrix is the chemical framework in a

foodstuff that binds together macro and micronutrients, fibre, water content and other bioactive substances. Understanding its composition and grid-like function is crucial to understanding the interactions between different components of foods, how they are digested and how they impact our health. Natural whole foods display a more pronounced food matrix than industrially processed foods, in which nutrients are typically only bound together by emulsifiers.

Macronutrients

Macronutrients are nutrients which the body requires in large quantities. The three main groups of macronutrients are carbohydrates, proteins and fats. Carbohydrates are long chains of sugars and supply the body with energy. They are abundant in grains, fruits and vegetables. Proteins are long chains of amino acids. They are the building blocks for cells, tissue and enzymes in both plants and animals. Meat, fish, dairy products and pulses are rich in proteins. Fats have a higher energy density and support the uptake of fat-soluble micronutrients. Fats are abundant in oils, nuts, seeds and avocados. However, the proportions of macronutrients in our food have proven surprisingly unimportant for a healthy diet, presumably because, in a healthy body, macronutrients are broken down and converted. Our bodies produce their own carbohydrates, proteins and fats in the necessary proportions.

Micronutrients

Micronutrients are nutrients that the body requires in small quantities, including vitamins (from fruits and vegetables), minerals such as calcium (from dairy products and green vegetables) and trace elements such as iron (found in meat and pulses) and zinc (from meat and nuts). Micronutrient deficiencies are rare in Western countries, but an excess of micronutrients may occur, mainly due to unregulated high-dose supplements. Nevertheless, significant micronutrient deficiencies do exist, for instance, among people suffering from severe eating and digestive disorders. Similarly, Vitamin D deficiency is common in young children and iodine deficiency is found in certain regions.

Nutritional energy

Nutritional energy is the amount of energy that the body receives from the consumption of foodstuffs. Nutrients such as carbohydrates, proteins and fats are major sources of nutritional energy. They are often indicated in kilocalories (kcal) or kilojoules (kJ). Nutritional energy is used by the body to regulate vital bodily functions, such as body temperature, organ function and physical activity. But nutritional energy also impacts mental processes and can be interpreted spiritually as a flow of energy within our bodies and between us and our environment. However, the body has difficulty disposing of excess energy from nutrients, which is why it is important to avoid overeating. Both body and mind need time and rest to relieve unnecessary physical and mental energy.

Nutri-Score

The Nutri-Score is a food labelling system intended to provide consumers with an overview of a product's nutritional quality (ranked from Green (A) to Red (E)). However, the Nutri-Score does not take the food matrix or the diversity of nutrients in a food into account. In addition, the food industry has exerted such a profound influence on the Nutri-Score over the years that industrially processed products now receive exceptionally positive ratings. For example, the cut-off point for added sugars is particularly high. As a result, consumers are better off following simple maxims like those from experts such as Tim Spector and Michael Pollan: 'Eat food. Not too much. Mostly plants.'

Serotonin, Tryptophan

Serotonin is a messenger substance in the central nervous system and gut which regulates mood, sleep and appetite. The serotonin-deficiency theory, which attributed depression to a lack of serotonin, is increasingly being debunked.

Tryptophan is an essential amino acid absorbed from food (such as poultry, dairy and nuts) and facilitates serotonin production in the brain and gut. However, studies examining whether tryptophan could be used to treat depression revealed no discernible effect, confirming the doubts cast on the theory of serotonin deficiency. In a world of excess, a lack of nutrients is an unlikely cause of the disease, but, as we know, overeating itself can increase the risk of non-communicable diseases, such as obesity, diabetes and autoimmune conditions.

Tube feeding, Parenteral feeding

Tube feeding is an artificial feeding method in which liquid nutrients are delivered directly into the stomach or intestines via a tube. It is considered necessary when a patient is deemed incapable of taking in sufficient food by mouth, as seen with swallowing disorders, eating disorders, or severe physical illnesses. This treatment requires the patient's gut to be able to digest the food.

Parenteral feeding is the practice of directly feeding nutrients into the bloodstream, typically via an intravenous catheter. This method is used when both eating and digestion are deemed impossible, or if parts of the gut are not functioning correctly. Patients receiving complete parenteral nutrition do not experience bowel movements.

The vagus nerve

The vagus nerve, also known as the tenth cranial nerve, is the longest nerve connecting the brain with internal organs such as the gut. It stretches from the brain, through the throat, to the abdomen. As part of the parasympathetic nervous system, which is responsible for soothing the body, relaxation, regeneration and digestion, the vagus nerve plays a crucial role in vital functions such as heart rate, breathing and digestion. It also influences mentally and socially significant processes such as mimicry and mood. Clinical studies also indicate that targeted stimulation of the vagus nerve can have therapeutic effects, reducing stress and benefiting mental health. Mindful eating and mindful toileting are among the most effective ways to activate the vagus nerve.

ENDNOTES

The Secret to a Good, Long Life

1.   Ives M, Ueno H, Inoue M. At 119, She Was a Symbol of How to Live with Wit and Vitality. *New York Times*. 2022.

2.   Santucci C, Mignozzi S, Malvezzi M, *et al.* European cancer mortality predictions for the year 2024 with focus on colo- rectal cancer. *Ann Oncol*. 2024.

3.   Conrad N, Misra S, Verbakel JY, *et al.* Incidence, prevalence, and co-occurrence of autoimmune disorders over time and by age, sex, and socioeconomic status: A population-based cohort study of 22 million individuals in the UK. *Lancet*. 2023; 401 (10391): 1878 – 1890.

4.   Buettner D, Skemp S. Blue Zones: Lessons from the world's longest lived. *Am J Lifestyle Med*. 2016; 10 (5): 318 – 321.

5.   Straznicky NE, Lambert EA, Lambert GW, Esler MD. Autonomic nervous system: Metabolic function. In: Reference *Module in Neuroscience and Biobehavioral Psychology*. 2017.

Mindful Eating

1.   Pinto JM, Wroblewski KE, Kern DW, Schumm LP, McClintock MK. Olfactory dysfunction predicts 5-year mortality in older adults. *PLoS One*. 2014; 9 (10): e107541.

2.   Receputo G, Mazzoleni G, Rapisarda R, *et al.* Sense of smell in centenarians from Eastern Sicily. *Arch Gerontol Geriatr*. 1996; 22 Suppl 1: 407 – 410.

3.   Alia S, Andrenelli E, Di Paolo A, Membrino V, Mazzanti L, Capecci M, *et al.* Chemosensory impairments and their im- pact on nutrition in Parkinson's disease: A narrative literature review. *Nutrients*. 2025;17(4):671. doi:10.3390/nu17040671. PMID: 40004999.

4.   Carriere K, Khoury B, Gunak MM, Knauper B. Mindfulness- based interventions for weight loss: A systematic review and meta-analysis. *Obes Rev*. 2018; 19 (2): 164 – 177.

5.   Park HD, Blanke O. Coupling inner and outer body for self-consciousness. *Trends Cogn Sci*. 2019; 23 (5): 377 – 388.

6.   Rochat P. What is it like to be a newborn? In: Gallagher S, ed. *The Oxford Handbook of the Self*. Oxford University Press. 2013.

7.   Blomkvist A, Hofer M. Olfactory impairment and close social relationships. A narrative review. *Chem Senses*. 2021; 46.

8.   Nijland R, Burgess JG. Bacterial olfaction. *Biotechnol J*. 2010; 5(9): 974 – 977

9. Force USPST, Mangione CM, Barry MJ, *et al.* Vitamin, Mineral, and multivitamin supplementation to prevent cardiovascular disease and cancer: US preventive services task force recommendation statement. *JAMA.* 2022; 327(23): 2326 – 2333.

10. Sandri A, Cecchini MP, Riello M, *et al.* Pain, Smell, and taste in adults: A narrative review of multisensory perception and interaction. *Pain Ther.* 2021; 10 (1): 245 – 268.

11. Drareni K, Dougkas A, Giboreau A, Laville M, Souquet PJ, Bensafi M. Relationship between food behavior and taste and smell alterations in cancer patients undergoing chemotherapy: A structured review. *Semin Oncol.* 2019; 46 (2): 160 – 172.

12. Vollmann-Profe G, von Magdeburg M. Das fließende Licht der Gottheit: Eine Auswahl. Mittelhochdeutsch/Neuhoch- deutsch. *Reclam.* 2008.

13. Reis DJ, Ilardi SS, Namekata MS, Wing EK, Fowler CH. The depressogenic potential of added dietary sugars. *Med Hypotheses.* 2020; 134: 109421.

14. Yang, Quanhe *et al.* 'Added sugar intake and cardiovascular diseases mortality among US adults.' *JAMA internal medicine.* vol. 174,4 (2014): 516-24. doi:10.1001/jamainternmed.2013.13563

15. Toews I, Lohner S, Küllenberg de Gaudry D, Sommer H, Meerpohl JJ. Association between intake of non-sugar sweeteners and health outcomes: Systematic review and meta- analyses of randomized and non-randomized controlled trials and observational studies. *BMJ.* 2019; 364: l156. doi:10.1136/bmj.l156. PMID: 30602577.

16. Mantantzis K, Schlaghecken F, Sunram-Lea SI, Maylor EA. Sugar rush or sugar crash? A meta-analysis of carbohydrate effects on mood. *Neurosci Biobehav Rev.* 2019; 101: 45 – 67.

17. Toda Y, Hayakawa T, Itoigawa A, *et al.* Evolution of the primate glutamate taste sensor from a nucleotide sensor. *Curr Biol.* 2021; 31 (20): 4641 – 4649 e4645.

18. James W, Skrupskelis IK, Berkeley EM. *The Correspondence of William James: April 1908-August 1910* (Volume 12). Uni- versity of Virginia Press. 2004.

19. Gupta DK, Lewis CE, Varady KA, *et al.* Effect of dietary sodium on blood pressure: A crossover trial. *JAMA.* 2023; 330 (23): 2258 – 2266.

20. PMID: 15962183: Abreu NP, Nunes DS, Oliveira LM, Francischetti EA. Effect of an isotonic rehydration sports drink and exercise on renal function in male Wistar rats. *Braz J Med Biol Res.* 2005; 38 (6): 869-875. doi:10.1590/S0100-879X2005000600009

21. Schwalfenberg GK. The alkaline diet: Is there evidence that an alkaline pH diet benefits health? *J Environ Public Health.* 2012; 2012: 727630.

22. Raposa B, Antal E, Macharia J, *et al.* The issue of acidity and alkalinity in our diet – Facts, popular beliefs, and the reality. *Acta Alimentaria.* 2022; 51(3): 326 – 340.

23. Breslin PAS. Interactions among salty, sour and bitter com- pounds. *Trends in Food Science & Technology.* 1996; 7 (12): 390 – 399.

24. Sagioglou C, Greitemeyer T. Individual differences in bitter taste preferences are associated with antisocial personality traits. *Appetite.* 2016; 96: 299 – 308.

25. Tian J, Geiss C, Zarse K, Madreiter-Sokolowski CT, Ristow M. Green tea catechins EGCG and ECG enhance the fitness and lifespan of Caenorhabditis elegans by complex I inhibition. *Aging* (Albany NY). 2021; 13(19): 22629 – 22648.

26. Allende I. *Aphrodite: A Memoir of the Senses.* HarperVia. 1999.

27. Moore J. *Fat Girl: A True Story.* Penguin. 2006.

28. Burton RF. *The Perfumed Garden of the Shaykh Nafzawi.* Independently published 2022.

29. Thich NH, Richard U. *Einfach essen.* O. W. Barth. 2016.

Microfasting and Macrofasting

1. PMID: 35627115; PMID: 38416492: Islam MR, Nyholt DR. Glucose-related traits and risk of migraine – A potential mechanism and treatment consideration. *Genes* (Basel). 2022; 13 (5): 730. doi:10.3390/genes13050730. PMID: 35627115; Heo GY, Koh HB, Park JT, Han SH, Yoo TH, Kang SW, Kim HW. Sweetened beverage intake and incident chronic kidney disease in the UK Biobank Study. *JAMA* Netw Open. 2024;7(2):e2356885. doi:10.1001/jamanetworkopen.2023.56885. PMID: 38416492.

2. Matarese G. The link between obesity and autoimmunity. *Science.* 2023; 379 (6639): 1298 – 1300

3. Hamsun K. *Hunger.* Projekt Gutenberg. 1921.

4. Climacus J. *The Ladder Of Divine Ascent: St. John Climacus* Translated by Archimandrite Lazarus Moore. Harper & Brothers. 1959.

5. Lau S, Hasler G. Nahrungsergänzungsmittel: Warum Vorsicht geboten ist. In: *Annabelle Magazin* Online. 2023.

6. Matarese G. The link between obesity and autoimmunity. *Science.* 2023; 379 (6639): 1298 – 1300.

7. Longo VD, Anderson RM. Nutrition, longevity and disease: From molecular mechanisms to interventions. *Cell.* 2022;185 (9): 1455 – 1470.

8. Hasler G, Buysse DJ, Klaghofer R, *et al.* The association bet- ween short sleep duration and obesity in young adults: A 13-year prospective study. *Sleep.* 2004; 27(4): 661 – 666.

Whole foods

1. Pollan M. *In Defense of Food: An Eater's Manifesto*. Penguin. 2008.

2. Sacks FM, Bray GA, Carey VJ, *et al*. Comparison of weight- loss diets with different compositions of fat, protein, and carbohydrates. *N Engl J Med*. 2009; 360 (9): 859 – 873.

3. PMID: 37341796: Martini D, da Costa Ribeiro H, Gately P, Mattes R, Re R, Bier D. Positive nutrition: Shifting the focus from nutrients to diet for a healthy lifestyle. *Eat Weight Disord*. 2023; 28(1): 51. doi:10.1007/s40519-023-01580-1.

4. Martini D, da Costa Ribeiro H, Gately P, Mattes R, Re R, Bier D. Positive nutrition: Shifting the focus from nutrients to diet for a healthy lifestyle. *Eat Weight Disord*. 2023; 28 (1): 51. doi: 10.1007/s40519-023-01580-1. PMID: 37341796

5. Smits SA, Leach J, Sonnenburg ED, *et al*. Seasonal cycling in the gut microbiome of the Hadza hunter-gatherers of Tanzania. *Science*. 2017; 357 (6353): 802 – 806.

6. Spector T. *Food for Life: The New Science of Eating Well*. Jonathan Cape. 2023.

7. Ali MK, Liu L, Chen JH, Huizinga JD. Optimizing autonomic function analysis via heart rate variability associated with motor activity of the human colon. *Front Physiol*. 2021; 12: 619722.

8. Englyst HN, Cummings JH. Digestion of the carbohydrates of banana (Musa paradisiaca sapientum) in the human small intestine. *Am J Clin Nutr*. 1986; 44 (1): 42 – 50.

9. Liu W, Jin Y, Wilde PJ, Hou Y, Wang Y, Han J. Mechanisms, physiology, and recent research progress of gastric emptying. *Crit Rev Food Sci Nutr*. 2021; 61 (16): 2742 – 2755.

10. Chassaing B, Koren O, Goodrich JK, *et al*. Dietary emulsifiers impact the mouse gut microbiota promoting colitis and metabolic syndrome. *Nature*. 2015; 519 (7541): 92 – 96.

11. Hecht EM, Layton MR, Abrams GA, Rhee JJ, Satija A, Rosner BA, Willett WC, Sun Q, Hu FB, Fung TT. Association of ultra-processed food consumption with risk of depression among older US adults: a prospective cohort study. *JAMA* Network Open. 2022; 5 (11): e2244491. doi: 10.1001/jamanetworkopen.2022.44491.

12. Nasi, S.; Romani, M.; Busso, N. Age-Associated Calcification: Insights from Murine Models. Gout Urate Cryst. *Depos. Dis.*, 2 (3), (2024), 236–251. https://doi.org/10.3390/gucdd2030018.

13. Liu Y, Nguyen M, Robert A, Meunier B. Metal ions in Alzheimer's disease: A key role or not? *Acc Chem Res*. 2019; 52 (7): 2026 – 2035.

14. Z He, Chang M, *et al*. Effects of Oral Vitamin C Supplemen- tation on Liver Health and Glucose Homeostasis. Antioxidants (Basel). 2021; 10 (12):1919. doi:10.3390/antiox10121919. PMID: 34798161; LeBoff MS, *et al*. Effects of Supplemental Vitamin D on Bone

Health Outcomes: A Systematic Review and Meta-analysis. J *Clin Endocrinol Metab*. 2020; 105 (4): e1049-1062. doi:10.1210/clinem/dgz216. PMID: 31971788; Allen JA, Peterson A, Sufit R, Varga J. Post-Epidemic Eosino- philia–Myalgia Syndrome Associated with L-Tryptophan. *Arthritis & Rheumatism*. 2011; 63 (3): 843-52. doi: 10.1002/art.30514. PMID: 21418049.

15. Nie C, Li Y, Qian H, Ying H, Wang L. Advanced glycation end products in food and their effects on intestinal tract. *Crit Rev Food Sci Nutr*. 2022; 62 (11): 3103 – 3115.

16. Mozaffarian D, Wu JH. Omega-3 fatty acids and cardio- vascular disease: effects on risk factors, molecular pathways, and clinical events. *J Am Coll Cardiol*. 2011; 58: 2047–67; Burr ML, Ashfield-Watt PA, Dunstan FD, Fehily AM, Breay P, Ashton T, *et al.* Lack of benefit of dietary advice to men with angina: results of a controlled trial. *Eur J Clin Nutr*. 2003; 57: 193–200.

17. Gould JF, Treyvaud K, Yelland LN, *et al.* Seven-year follow-up of children born to women in a randomized trial of prenatal DHA supplementation. *JAMA*. 2017;317(11): 1173 – 1175.

18. Okereke OI, Vyas CM, Mischoulon D, *et al.* Effect of long- term supplementation with marine omega-3 fatty acids vs placebo on risk of depression or clinically relevant depressive symptoms and oncChange in mood scores: A randomized clinical trial. *JAMA*. 2021; 326 (23): 2385 – 2394.

19. Eberli F. Omega-3-Fettsäuren: Chronischer Hype ohne Evidenz? *Swiss Medical Forum*. 2023; 23(17):1026 – 1030.

20. Goethe J; Auden W. H.; Mayer E. *Italian Journey*. Penguin Classics. 1992.

21. McDonald D, Hyde E, Debelius JW, Morton JT, Gonzalez A, Ackermann G, *et al.* American Gut: An open platform for citizen science microbiome research. *mSystems*. 2018; 3 (3): e00031-18. doi:10.1128/mSystems.00031-18. PMID: 29795809.

22. Wastyk HC, Fragiadakis GK, Perelman D, *et al.* Gut-microbiota-targeted diets modulate human immune status. Cell. 2021; 184(16): 4137-4153.e14.

23. Olivelle P. *Upanisads*. Oxford University Press. 2008.

24. Nikolova VL, Cleare AJ, Young AH, Stone JM. Acceptability, tolerability, and estimates of putative treatment effects of probiotics as adjunctive treatment in patients with depression: A randomized clinical trial. *JAMA* psychiatry. 2023; 80 (8): 842 – 847.

25. Concas MP, Morgan A, Tesolin P, Santin A, Girotto G, Gasparini P. Sensory capacities and eating behavior: Intriguing results from a large cohort of Italian individuals. *Foods*. 2022; 11 (5).

Eating Rituals and Eating in Company

1. Hasuo H, Kusaka N, Sano M, *et al.* Effects of eating toget- her online on autonomic nervous system functions: A ran- domized, open-label, controlled preliminary study among healthy volunteers. *Biopsychosoc Med.* 2023; 17 (1): 10.

2. The first parliaments in Europe were known as 'diets', such as the 'Diéta' of the Habsburg Empire. The word 'diet' was mistakenly associated with the Latin 'dies', meaning 'day'. This gave rise to the German term 'Bundestag', which should really be called the 'Bundesdiät'. The correct term would have had the advantage of reminding us that political activity is not simply a matter of having meetings; it is about fair distribution to and healthy nourishment of the people.

3. Gregersen SC, Gillath O. How food brings us together: The ties between attachment and food behaviors. *Appetite.* 2020; 151: 104654.

4. Petzold A, van den Munkhof HE, Figge-Schlensok R, Korotkova T. Complementary lateral hypothalamic popu- lations resist hunger pressure to balance nutritional and social needs. *Cell Metab.* 2023; 35 (3): 456 – 471 e456.

5. Dunbar RIM. Breaking bread: The functions of social eating. *Adapt Human Behav Physiol.* 2017; 3 (3): 198 – 211.

6. *Ibid.*

7. Johnson, Katerina V.-A. 'Gut Microbiome Composition and Diversity Are Related to Human Personality Traits'. *Human Microbiome Journal*, vol. 15, 2020, article 100069, https://doi.org/10.1016/j.humic.2019.100069.

8. Gacesa R, Kurilshikov A, Vich Vila A, *et al.* Environmental factors shaping the gut microbiome in a Dutch population. *Nature.* 2022; 604 (7907): 732 – 739.

9. Allende I. *Aphrodite: A Memoir of the Senses.* HarperVia. 1999.

10. Kügler J. Die Macht der Nase. *Zur religiösen Bedeutung des Duftes.* Vol 187. Verlag Katholisches Bibelwerk.

11. Rageot M, Hussein RB, Beck S, *et al.* Biomolecular analyses enable new insights into ancient Egyptian embalming. *Nature.* 2023; 614 (7947): 287 – 293.

12. Farb P, Armelagos G. *Consuming Passions: The Anthropology of Eating.* Houghton Mifflin Harcourt. 198

Transforming nutritional energy

1. Prabhavananda S, Isherwood C, Huxley A. *Bhagavad-Gita: The Song of God.* Signet. 2002.

2. Thich Nhat Hanh. *How to Eat.* Illustrated by Jason DeAntonis. Berkeley: Parallax Press, 2014

Cleansing

1. McCracken C, Raisi-Estabragh Z, Veldsman M, *et al.* Multi- organ imaging demonstrates the heart-brain-liver axis in UK Biobank participants. *Nature communications.* 2022; 13 (1): 7839.

2. Tucci M, Marino M, Martini D, Porrini M, Riso P, Del Bo C. Plant-based foods and vascular function: A systematic review of dietary intervention trials in older subjects and hypothesized mechanisms of action. *Nutrients.* 2022; 14 (13).

3. Jang Y, Nyamjav I, Kim HR, *et al.* Identification of plastic- degrading bacteria in the human gut. *Sci Total Environ.* 2024; 929: 172775.

4. Hill W, Lim EL, Weeden CE, *et al.* Lung adenocarcinoma promotion by air pollutants. *Nature.* 2023; 616 (7955): 159–167.

5. Asnicar F, Leeming ER, Dimidi E, *et al.* Blue poo: impact of gut transit time on the gut microbiome using a novel marker. *Gut.* 2021; 70 (9): 1665 – 1674.

6. Critchley HOD, Babayev E, Bulun SE, *et al.* Menstruation: Science and society. *Am J Obstet Gynecol.* 2020; 223 (5): 624 – 664.

7. Hildegard & Berger, M. (1999) *On natural philosophy and medicine: selections from Cause et cure.* Cambridge: D.S. Brewer.

8. Hasler G, Buysse DJ, Klaghofer R, *et al.* The association between short sleep duration and obesity in young adults: A 13-year prospective study. *Sleep.* 2004; 27 (4): 661 – 666.

9. Xie L, *et al.* (2013) 'Sleep drives metabolite clearance from the adult brain.' *Science.* 342 (6156): 373 – 377

10. Klinzing JG, Niethard N, Born J. Mechanisms of systems memory consolidation during sleep. *Nat Neurosci.* 2019; 22 (10): 1598 – 1610.

11. Withrow D, Bowers SJ, Depner CM, González A, Reynolds AC, Wright KP Jr. Sleep and circadian disruption and the gut microbiome – Possible links to dysregulated metabolism. *Curr Opin Endocr Metab Res.* 2021; 17: 26-37. doi:10.1016/j.coemr.2020.11.009. PMID: 34805616.

12. TuSmith B. *All My Relatives: Community in Contemporary Ethnic American Literature.* University of Michigan Press. 1994.

13. Okakura, Kakuzō. *The Book of Tea.* Culturea, 2023. Originally published 1906.

THANKS

I want to thank Paolo Gasparini, Catherine Maher, Andreas Luft from the Lake Lucerne Institute in Vitznau, and Dragos Inta at the University of Freiburg, Switzerland, for their scientific and neuronutritive inspiration while writing this book. I would also like to thank Daniela Roth, Marc Germann, Hannelore Daniel, Morten Lietz, Simon Duttwyler, Pascal Pompetzki, Svenja Liebschner and Christina Keinath for their valuable pointers on food, cooking and digestion. I want to thank my mother, Theri Hasler, Janine Antonov and David Simeon, for their invaluable and stimulating comments on the manuscript. I also want to thank Stéphanie Majerus, Jens Schlieter, Barbara Schweizer and Samuel Vollenweider for drawing my attention to the spiritual and ritualistic aspects of fasting, cooking and eating, and Simon Küpfer for pointing out the etymological origins of the word 'diet'. I'd also like to thank Caroline Colsman, Stella Christiansen, and Stephanie Taverna from Arkana Verlag for their expertise and enthusiasm.

Gregor Hasler is Professor of Psychiatry and Psycho-therapy at the *University of Fribourg*, specialising in the relationship between nutrition and mental health. Following a three-year research fellowship at the *National Institute of Mental Health* (USA), his current research focuses on eating behaviours, the gut-brain axis and the impact of nutrition on emotional resilience. An internationally recognised speaker on eating disorders, depression and nutritional psychiatry, his ground-breaking cohort studies explore how dietary habits and the microbiome influence psychological states. Winner of the prestigious *Robert Bing Prize* from the *Swiss Academy of Medical Sciences*, Professor Hasler bridges cutting-edge science with practical guidance, helping readers understand how food shapes both physical and mental well-being.

Dr Janette Walton is an esteemed academic, currently serving as a Senior Lecturer in Biological Sciences and Head of the NutRI research group at Munster Technological University in Ireland. With over thirty years' experience spanning industry and academia in food, nutrition and health, Dr Walton's primary research interests are in the dietary habits of the Irish population across the lifecycle. She has published more than 100 research papers in this area and serves on advisory committees in nutrition and food, both nationally and internationally.

Ayça Türkoğlu is a writer and translator from Turkish and German into English. She co-translated Selim Özdoğan's *Anatolian Blues* trilogy from German. Her work has been shortlisted for the Helen & Kurt Wolff Translator's Prize. She lives in North London.